Better Communication for Better Care

To my wife, Diane L. Stowe-Cohn, whose encouragement, love, and outstanding family nurturing made writing this book not only possible but also pleasurable.

To my children, Livie and Peter Cohn, (continue to) teach your parents well.

Your board, staff, or clients may also benefit from this book's insight. For more information on quantity discounts, contact the Health Administration Press Marketing Manager at (312) 424-9470.

This publication is intended to provide accurate and authoritative information in regard to the subject matter covered. It is sold, or otherwise provided, with the understanding that the publisher is not engaged in rendering professional services. If professional advice or other expert assistance is required, the services of a competent professional should be sought.

The statements and opinions contained in this book are strictly those of the author(s) and do not represent the official positions of the American College of Healthcare Executives or of the Foundation of the American College of Healthcare Executives.

09 08 07 06 05   5 4 3 2 1

Library of Congress Cataloging-in-Publication Data

Cohn, Kenneth H.
    Better communication for better care : mastering physician-administrator collaboration / Kenneth H. Cohn.
        p. cm.
    Includes bibliographical references.
    ISBN 1-56793-238-X (alk. paper)
    1. Hospitals—Medical staff. 2. Hospitals—Administration. 3. Hospital-physician relations. I. Title.

RA972.C56 2005
610.69'6—dc22

                                                                    2004060902

The paper used in this publication meets the minimum requirements of American National Standard for Information Sciences—Permanence of Paper for Printed Library Materials, ANSI Z39.48-1984. ∞ ™

Acquisitions editor: Audrey Kaufman; Project manager: Joyce Sherman; Layout editor: Amanda Karvelaitis; Cover design: Trisha Lartz

Health Administration Press
A division of the Foundation of the
    American College of Healthcare Executives
1 North Franklin Street, Suite 1700
Chicago, IL 60606-4425
(312) 424-2800

Introduction

The premise of this book is that physicians and hospital leaders, including senior executives and midlevel managers, working interdependently can achieve more than either group could working independently. This goal is challenging for both groups because of differences in culture and training and because current incentives have not facilitated interdependence. Cost-based reimbursement previously allowed both groups to pass on cost increases regardless of inefficiency and duplication of services. The current economic climate has exacerbated differences in outlook and training as financial pressures create strains over how to divide what feels like a fixed or shrinking pie.

From a community perspective, both physicians and hospital leaders care for the same patients, have complementary skills, and waste scarce resources by working independently rather than interdependently. Working harder doing the same activities but expecting different results is not a practical solution. New ways of interacting merit consideration.

This book is written from my perspective as both a physician and a patient (having survived lymphoma), and it applies to healthcare workers interested in working more productively to improve their care and service to patients.

If we agree that physicians and hospital leaders practice in a symbiotic environment, physicians need to learn about a variety of issues for which they have received little or no training in medical school, residency, or fellowship. Project-based, just-in-time learning, for example, gives physicians the background information they need to understand issues when medicine and business intersect as part of a clinically based undertaking at the appropriate time.

It is difficult for physicians and hospital leaders to admit that they do not have all the answers precisely because so many people rely on them for answers. Yet responding, "I do not know. What do you think?" can lead to richer, more productive solutions and improve employee morale and retention.

In writing this book, I am aware that neither physicians nor healthcare executives are homogeneous and that each profession attracts a variety of personalities. I hope that despite their differences, physicians and hospital leaders who are willing to entertain new ideas can make their time count, their service productive, and their legacy lasting.

CHAPTER 1

The Structured Dialogue Process

Kenneth H. Cohn

"**W**hatever you do, you know that we will return to our usual ways after you leave, so why don't you save the hospital money and save us time and leave now?" replied a skeptical surgeon when asked for his opinion about a proposed consulting engagement at the hospital where he worked. The consultant asked this surgeon what he recommended to obtain physicians' collaboration in clinical improvement efforts at his hospital. The surgeon responded, "The solution is simple. If you get us [physicians] in a room together, we are naked in front of our peers. We may pay lip service to administrators, but we tell the truth to people who we refer patients to and who refer patients to us. "▶

INTRODUCTION

Hospital executives quip that the most expensive device in U.S. hospitals is the physician's pen. The hospital is a derivative business in that physicians greatly influence clinical revenues, expenses, and outcomes by their decision making (Larson 2002). Because of the different ways that physicians and administrators tend to view decision making, previous attempts to involve physicians in hospital processes have created conflicts that have worsened physician-administrator relationships. Physicians tend to be more entrepreneurial, independent, and task focused than executives, who tend to be more deliberate, consensus oriented, and organizationally focused (Gill 1987; Cohn, Gill, and Schwartz 2005). Physicians have clinical expertise but lack experience in administrative affairs and thus feel that administrators dominate hospital meetings. Both sides talk at each other without fully appreciating or understanding the other's concerns. The meetings are built on the false assumption that "alignment" is the goal and therefore fail to address those physician issues that differ from and may be in conflict with those of the hospital. The challenge is to find common ground while acknowledging differences.

As physicians have grown busier, hospitalists have provided inpatient care, and primary care physicians may not even set foot in hospitals except for social visits. An unfortunate consequence is that physicians spend less time in face-to-face interactions with colleagues and thus grow distant from one another. When physician-physician communication and collaboration are lacking, physician-administration communication suffers because physicians do not reach consensus on a collective self-interest regarding hospital operations and optimal care for the community. Structured dialogue offers a potential win-win approach by improving physician-administration and physician-physician communication. The purpose of this chapter is to describe the structured dialogue process and to delineate the prerequisites for success.

WHAT IS STRUCTURED DIALOGUE?

Structured dialogue is a process that helps a group of physicians to articulate its collective, patient-centered self-interest. For example, structured dialogue can help physicians establish clinical priorities for the next three to five years. The structured dialogue process is led by a panel of high-performing, well-respected clinicians, who review and recommend clinical priorities based on presentations by the major clinical sections and departments. The clinical priorities are presented in a report that contains a statement of the direction in which the hospital should be heading, rather than a list of capital-intensive budget items. In return for giving physicians a say in clinical priority setting, the hospital is able to enlist physicians to attend meetings and outline their priorities.

Value Proposition

For administrators interested in developing physician engagement and a sense of ownership among their medical staff and decreasing the cost and variability of medical care, structured dialogue is valuable in the following ways:

- It addresses issues such as revenues, costs, financial collaboration, clinical services, and clinical outcomes.
- It creates an environment in which physicians are willing to be accountable to one another and

open to facilitating long-term change.
- It helps channel hospital investments into high-priority services based on community needs and clinical strengths.
- It creates an ongoing forum for open and effective dialogue among physicians and hospital leaders.
- It facilitates solutions to service problems that do not require major capital expenditures.
- It identifies and develops new physician leaders.

Implementation Method

Figure 1 represents the process that has been used over the past 15 years by Cambridge Management Group to maximize physicians' and administrators' effectiveness while respecting individual differences in hospital size, location, and culture (Cohn 2002).

Process. The process begins by one-on-one and small group meetings with practicing physicians to ascertain their willingness to work together to improve medical care for the community. If they are willing, the chief executive officer (CEO) and board agree to alter their approach to strategic planning to allow the physicians approximately six months for presentations, discussion, and

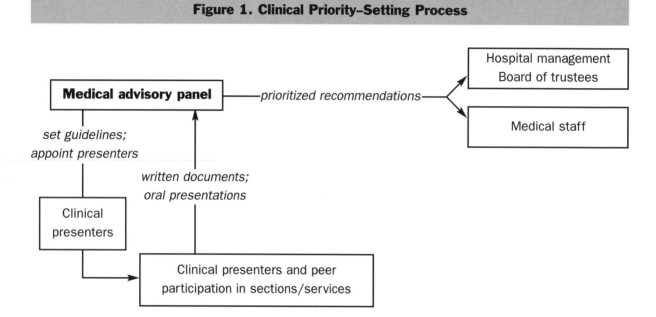

Figure 1. Clinical Priority–Setting Process

Medical advisory panel ——prioritized recommendations——

Hospital management
Board of trustees

Medical staff

set guidelines;
appoint presenters

written documents;
oral presentations

Clinical
presenters

Clinical presenters and peer
participation in sections/services

Source: Cohn (2002). Reprinted courtesy of the American College of Physician Executives.

report writing. Next, the CEO, in consultation with physician leaders, appoints two cochairs based on their clinical ability, the level of respect of their colleagues, and their leadership ability. The cochairs pick the remainder of the medical advisory panel (MAP) based on similar criteria. A time line for this process used recently at a community teaching hospital is shown in Figure 2.

MAP agenda. During its first meeting, the MAP picks physician presenters from all major departments and clinical sections. The physician presenters meet with their department or section members; develop consensus on their needs and concerns; and give written and oral presentations on the strengths, weaknesses, opportunities, and threats (also known as a SWOT analysis) facing their clinical areas. The reports generally list five consensus-based recommendations as their top clinical priorities.

Report writing. The MAP evaluates presenters' recommendations based on their potential to improve care, communication, and revenue and to reduce costs. It then writes a report

Figure 2. Clinical Priority–Setting Process Time Line

Project Schedule

Month 1	Month 2	Month 3
Project design and organization	MAP operations	Section presentations

Select cochairs, panel

1st working sessions

Information gathering

Briefing section presenters

Two section presentations per week

Month 4	Month 5	Month 6
Section presentations	Presentations/ analysis	MAP report

Two section presentations per week

MAP evaluates recommendations

Sets priorities for themes, initiatives

Cochairs draft final report

Review with MAP

Submit to
—physicians
—management
—board

Months 7–10: Implementation assistance to ensure effective realization of outcomes outlining major themes and recommendations. Fellow physicians, administrators, and board members read and discuss the report, come to consensus on priorities for implementation, and set the implementation timetable and assignment of responsibilities, as discussed below in the case study.

CASE STUDY

A 425-bed community teaching hospital in New England experienced a 10 percent clinical operating loss despite numerous cycles of reengineering and rapid-sequence change processes. After several months of discussion, the hospital and medical staff committed to the structured dialogue process. They formed a MAP because both the hospital and the physicians felt that practicing physicians needed a voice in determining clinical priorities over the next three years.

The hospital CEO and the vice president of medical affairs led the process of convening the MAP by selecting the cochairs based on their clinical ability and on the respect that they enjoyed with their peers. The cochairs in turn selected 11 other panel members based on clinical

ability, leadership skills, and credibility with peers.

To develop its recommendations, the MAP solicited input from the medical staff through a series of meetings and presentations with each clinical department and section. The MAP asked each clinical area to present its goals, long-term strategy, and short-term tactics. To support the clinical areas in developing their presentations, the hospital provided support staff and financial and demographic data, as requested. The MAP met weekly for four months to hear presentations from all major clinical departments and sections. The first presentation occurred approximately one month after the MAP convened, allowing time for MAP members and presenters to obtain necessary background information on hospital operations, nursing, marketing, finance, information services, and managed care contracting.

Clinical Priorities
Written and oral section reports allowed the MAP to weigh priorities. The panel incorporated the following four overarching themes into a written report:

1. Improve service to patients and families.

2. Enhance physician-to-physician communication.
3. Implement clinical protocols in all major diagnostic-related groups to save money, limit variation, and improve quality and safety.
4. Develop coordinated diagnostic and treatment centers.

These four themes were presented to the medical executive officers and staff, to senior management and department chairs, and to the board of trustees.

To outsiders, the themes might be considered mundane. For the hospital and physicians, however, obtaining consensus on these issues was a major achievement because physicians had not embraced these themes previously. Once the MAP concluded its initial report, administrator-physician teams worked to implement the MAP's recommendations over the next two years. The MAP reconvened quarterly to monitor the status of implementation, and several of the physicians from the MAP were involved in implementing the initiatives, as discussed below. Since implementation of the MAP recommendations, there has been a renewed emphasis on patient satisfaction, and surgical volumes and market share have increased, especially in minimally invasive cardiac surgery.

Implementation Efforts

The CEO and his senior administrative team met weekly to review and improve service to patients and families, resolving to change their competitive strategy from that of a high-tech hospital with the latest devices to that of a technologically advanced community hospital that emphasized service. Patient care managers were expected to make daily rounds and be proactive rather than reactive in improving service. A patient relations department was established, and the entire staff was educated on customer service techniques.

Medical staff departments were charged with the responsibility to update the medical staff on new developments, programs, and services at their quarterly staff meetings. Physicians felt that face-to-face contact improved physician-physician communication far more than sending out newsletters that few people made time to read. One improvement implemented was having consulting physicians fax their evaluations to requesting physicians within 24 hours rather than making physicians wait for a mailed letter.

Physicians also developed protocols that provided improved results quickly, such as a protocol for heparinized patients that decreased pages to physicians from the nurses and improved outcomes and a post-anesthesia recovery unit extubation protocol that cut overnight stays by one-third. They then built on those successes to develop consensus in more controversial areas, such as computerized physician order entry. A coordinated diagnostic and treatment center for patients with gastrointestinal complaints was under construction at the time of this writing.

Both management and physicians felt that the structured dialogue guided by the MAP achieved the following:

- Provided a stepwise process that improved the way that physicians related to their colleagues and served their community
- Put leadership for clinical direction back in the hands of physicians, and gave physicians a constructive way to make their voices heard
- Provided an innovative approach to strategic and operational planning based on physician guidance that changed the hospital's strategy from being a high-tech center to being a technologically advanced community hospital known for its service to patients and their families
- Provided an excellent approach for grooming the 13 physician leaders who served on the MAP by broadening their focus beyond their specialties

PREREQUISITES FOR SUCCESS

Two steps are required to help ensure successful implementation of the structured dialogue process. First, the hospital, board, and physicians must communicate in a clear, straightforward, effective manner.

- The hospital staff assists physicians as needed, realizing that the dialogue and recommendations may not fit the current hospital business model.
- The CEO and board, admitting that they lack physicians' clinical knowledge, give serious consideration to MAP recommendations for physicians to be willing to commit time as presenters and panelists.
- Physicians recognize their interdependency and responsibility

to one another and to the hospital and community.

■ Physicians maintain confidentiality during and after MAP presentations to avoid leaks of sensitive or proprietary data and to allow members to think aloud without fear of embarrassment.

Second, dialogue and recommendations must be comprehensive.

■ Consensus is required; no minority department or section reports are allowed.
■ The first priority remains the patient care needs of the community.

KEY CONCEPTS

■ Effective communication between physicians and administrators can yield an improved work environment and competitive advantage in a rapidly changing marketplace.

■ Physicians need an environment in which they can communicate on a peer-peer basis and define their collective priorities to be able to communicate more effectively with hospital leaders.

■ Hospital executives benefit from physician consensus on programmatic spending and process improvement.

REFERENCES

Cohn, K. H. 2002. "The Structured Dialogue Process." [Online article; retrieved 10/28/04.] *Click: The Online Journal of the American College of Physician Executives.* http://www.acpe.org/click /archive/index.cfm?fuseaction = display&ID = 77.

Cohn, K. H., S. L. Gill, and R. W. Schwartz. 2005. "Gaining Hospital Administrators' Attention: Ways to Improve Physician-Hospital Management Dialogue—A Case Report." *Surgery* 137 (2), in press.

Gill, S. L. 1987. "Can Doctors and Administrators Work Together?" *Physician Executive* 13 (5): 11–6.

Larson L. 2002. "Balance of Power: Encouraging Physicians to Help Set the Strategic Plan." *Trustee* September: 13–17.

CHAPTER 2

The Spectrum of Physician-Management Financial Collaboration

Kenneth H. Cohn and Thomas R. Allyn

"We need more than warm fuzzies to get in bed with the hospital," said a New Jersey cardiologist. Other cardiologists sitting around the table nodded their heads in agreement. In response to financial pressure created by rising expenses and stagnating reimbursement and increasing desire for efficiency and control of their schedules, physicians are performing procedures and services in outpatient settings that used to be done in hospitals. ▶

INTRODUCTION

The goal of physician-hospital financial collaboration is to create something of value that benefits patients, physicians, and the hospital. Collaboration implies win-win agreements that enlarge the economic pie rather than dividing decreasing shares. Both parties gain if physicians act as owners rather than clients, increasing admissions and revenue and collaborating on ways to improve processes and outcomes. The purpose of this chapter is to discuss opportunities for financial collaboration between physicians and hospital leaders and to recommend policies and procedures that will facilitate success.

FINANCIAL COLLABORATION OPPORTUNITIES

As outlined in Table 1, a spectrum of opportunities permits physicians and hospitals to partner in multiple ways. Beginning communication with

Table 1. Possible Physician-Hospital Collaboration Opportunities

Service Contracts	Lease/ Purchase	Contractual Integration	Subordinated Bonds	Joint Equity Ventures
Physician panels (e.g., electrocardiogram interpretation)	Physician office complex	Hospital within a hospital (e.g., orthopedic, cardiac, oncology, intensive care unit)	Ambulatory surgical center	Ambulatory surgical center
Medical directorships	Imaging center		Specialty hospital	Specialty hospital
	Cardiovascular diagnostic center		Cardiovascular imaging and treatment center	Regional center of excellence (e.g., neuroscience, cardiovascular, gastrointestinal, oncology)
Physician service contracts (e.g., pathology, emergency department, anesthesiology)	Cardiac catheterization laboratory			
Trauma stipends				

smaller projects may allow both parties to lay the groundwork for larger deals in the future. For example, service contracts pay physicians for interpreting diagnostic tests like electrocardiograms and for taking trauma call. Lease-purchase agreements allow physicians to build equity in office settings. Contractual integration, subordinated bonds, and joint equity deals permit physicians and hospitals to run specialty hospital facilities and ambulatory surgical centers together. Strengths and weaknesses of contractual integration, subordinated bonds, and joint equity ventures are outlined in Table 2.

Contractual integration creates a business entity within a hospital with an executive management council composed of eight to ten physicians and the hospital CEO or designate (Zismer and Burke 2003). Physicians receive compensation for providing patient care, developing and reviewing programs, and achieving nonfinancial milestones (to avoid violation of Stark laws, which prohibit rewards for referrals).

Subordinated bond deals involve purchase of tax-exempt bonds whose return varies with economic performance. Through a management service organization, physicians can obtain control of daily operations that affect their income, such as scheduling, personnel, and hours of operation. In addition, nonspecialist physicians are encouraged to invest. Because the surplus from these investments generates no taxable income for the hospital, the hospital retains its tax-exempt status and physician investors can enjoy higher rates of return (Cohn et al. 2005).

In *joint equity ventures*, the hospital and physicians own stock representing a facility, equipment, and personnel. Current tax laws place hospitals at a disadvantage in regard to joint equity ventures relative to outside promoters who build specialty hospitals or ambulatory surgical centers because, to retain its not-for-profit status, a charity must do the following:

■ Receive compensation for intangible assets (such as patients) transferred to the venture, usually at five to eight times the net income, creating a debt burden for the joint venture and making physicians feel as though the hospital is cheating them out of income from their private patients (Reeder 2003)
■ Have numerical control of the board of any joint venture, which can trigger physician discontent
■ Not refuse service to any category of patients (this is clearly not the

Table 2. Potential Strengths and Weaknesses of Financial Collaboration Models

Model	Strengths	Weaknesses
Contractual integration	Contract based No equity transferred	Relatively new No ownership of stock Limited room for outside investors
Subordinated bonds	Debt based No equity transferred No need to limit investors	Relatively new No ownership of stock Less liquid than municipal bonds
Joint equity venture	Stock based Potential for high return	Higher operating costs due to payment of property, sales, and income taxes Limited room for outside investors due to dilution Possible credit risk for hospitals*

* Moody's Investors Service asserts that the risks to hospitals of joint equity ventures, including loss of patient volume and revenue, creation of an indirect debt obligation, and potential for alienating physicians not allowed to invest (e.g., primary care physicians) generally outweigh the benefits (Moody's 2001).

Source: Cohn et al. (2005).

case if physicians choose to invest without the hospital) (Cohn et al. 2005)

RECOMMENDATIONS

It would be impractical to recommend one method of financial collaboration over another because each hospital community has different needs, culture, and risk tolerance. This chapter offers a snapshot of the possibilities in a dynamic, evolving setting. Building the transparency and trust necessary for success is a process in which progress is not linear and expectations need to be communicated, clarified, and revised on an ongoing basis. Therefore, we encourage potential investors on both sides to take the following steps:

- Ask "What if..." often in the early stages of discussion to learn more about each other's goals, needs, and expectations.
- Work proactively to develop a shared vision for the enterprise that will
  - improve care for the community;
  - allow the hospital to remain financially viable and to be in a position to invest for the future; and
  - rapidly identify and remove system roadblocks to effective and efficient care, which is key to retaining physician loyalty.
- Obtain counsel from attorneys who specialize in healthcare transactions.

KEY CONCEPTS

Successful physician-hospital financial collaboration requires the following:

- Mutual understanding of each party's interests and needs
- Sharing information widely
- Distinguishing thinking aloud from negotiating

- Stepwise building of transparency and trust, starting from scratch and not assuming agreement where none exists

- Both sides acting as a team of active owners rather than as individual, passive investors, jointly improving care processes in an ongoing fashion

REFERENCES

Cohn, K. H., T. R. Allyn, R. Rosenfield, and R. Schwartz. 2005. "Overview of Physician Ventures." *American Journal of Surgery*, in press.

Moody's Investors Service. 2001. "Hospital-Physician Joint Ventures: Credit Risks Generally Outweigh Benefits." Report No. 71717, November 1–4.

Reeder, L. 2003. "Exploring a New Alternative to Hospital/Physician Joint Ventures." *Healthcare Leadership & Management Report* 11 (2): 1–5.

Zismer, D. K., and F. G. Burke. 2003. "Contractual Integration: An Alternative to Equity-based Models for Hospital-Physician Specialty Services Partnerships." *Discovery* September: 1–12.

CHAPTER 3

When Physicians Compete with the Hospital

Kenneth H. Cohn and Thomas R. Allyn

"**N**obody cares what the hospital administration is thinking," growled a Mid-Atlantic general surgeon who formed an independent ambulatory surgical center. "Patients go where their docs tell them to go!" ▶

INTRODUCTION

Little has changed since Gill (1987) wrote about the tension between physicians and hospital administrators. We doubt that physicians and healthcare leaders were ever in alignment; what is different now, however, is that neither party can pass on cost increases independently of the other as happened previously. Like it or not, they are bound together in a complex web of interdependence.

As mentioned in Chapter 1, because most physicians' incomes derive from direct patient care and procedures rather than salary, they tend to be more entrepreneurial, independent, and task focused than healthcare executives, who tend to be more deliberate, consensus oriented, and organizationally focused (Gill 1987). The purpose of this chapter is to offer a three-part strategy of proactivity, collaborative conflict, and containment as a guide to dealing with physician-hospital competition. We empathize with the difficulty of predicting how events will unfold because the process requires faith that both parties will become stronger by loosening individual control.

PROACTIVITY

Physicians and hospital administrators need to discuss ways to collaborate in a proactive fashion. It may seem counterintuitive for leaders to take the lead in partnering with their highest-revenue-generating physicians, but a proactive approach minimizes the opportunity for external turnkey operators to create unrealistic expectations among physicians. Organizations outside the hospital that charge physicians a percentage of gross revenue can appear to provide heightened reimbursement to physicians who are unschooled in financial statement analysis. In turn, a more content medical staff can help the hospital and the community by decreasing the costs of clinical care and improving outcomes. As a rationale for talking with physicians proactively, following are some examples of what hospital executives can offer:

- Access to capital at a lower rate of interest than physicians generally can obtain on their own
- Participation advantages in the purchase of expensive, rapidly changing, high-tech equipment (e.g., computed tomography and magnetic resonance imaging scanners)
- Market power to obtain bundled reimbursement from payers for cutting-edge services
- Access to land near the hospital that it owns

- Experience with regulatory agencies related to certificate of need, zoning issues, and compliance with Stark and antikickback laws
- A known identity for patients that can provide comfort, security, and credibility

Collaboration succeeds when hospital leaders and physicians make effective dialogue a high priority and work closely together toward a common purpose. They can share information more productively if they understand exactly what each party needs and at what time intervals. We know of no better way to make information sharing a reality than if senior executives engage in periodic, face-to-face dialogue with their most productive physicians, regardless of their irascibility (Cohn, Gill, and Schwartz 2005). Items for discussion may include the following:

- Hospital issues that the physician would like to solve, the priority level of those issues, who at the hospital to contact about them, any roadblocks, and a timetable for reaching a solution
- Issues that the hospital would like to solve with the physician, the priority level of those issues, and a timetable for reaching a solution
- Information that the physician needs from the hospital, its format

(electronic or printed), and its frequency
- Information that the hospital needs from the physician (e.g., vacation dates, recruitment and succession plans)
- The physician's preferred mode of routine communication (i.e., in person, telephone, electronic) and the frequency
- Best times to meet and best settings for productive communication

Finding ways to communicate effectively may be difficult initially, but preliminary discussions help both parties discover what combination of activities works, ranging from breakfast meetings and chats between procedures to traveling to local or distant conferences together. The most important aspect is that communication efforts start now rather than in response to a crisis or waiting until an event in the distant future.

COLLABORATIVE CONFLICT

Conflict involves differences between people who believe that their feelings, thoughts, or actions are incompatible (Porter 1996). Conflict is inevitable in rapidly changing settings and therefore is neither positive nor negative; it is the response to conflict that determines whether the outcome is positive or negative (Lussier 1995).

In *collaborative conflict*, people attack problems rather than one another to solve them in a way that satisfies both parties and builds long-term relationships. Success depends on each party's preparation for and understanding of what each wants and needs to accomplish, what each is willing to concede, and which "hot buttons" might cause an angry response (Umiker 1997).

Hot Buttons

Active listening requires both parties to pay attention to body language and tone of voice, suspend judgment, clarify and summarize issues to the satisfaction of the other party, and be conscious of the effect of language. Avoiding accusatory inferences and inflammatory words, such as "you," "but," "always," "never," "I disagree," and "why," may help parties come to agreement. Similarly, initial brainstorming about the potential advantages of new approaches rather than focusing on potential obstacles, like costs, may help sustain fledgling discussions. In *Getting Past No*, Ury (1991) recommends a five-step approach to difficult negotiations.

1. *"Going to the balcony,"* allowing one to escape mentally to clarify thoughts about both parties' interests and reflect on the next steps
2. *Stepping aside*, akin to emotional jujitsu, enabling one to listen, acknowledge, defuse anger, and find areas of agreement on which to build
3. *Reframing*, letting the problem be the teacher, to foster a team-based approach with phrases such as, "What would you recommend to help us solve this problem?"
4. *Building bridges*, allowing both sides to save face and satisfy mutual interests
5. *Making it difficult to say no*, helping to decrease the risk of failure and reassuring each other that the goal is mutual satisfaction rather than unilateral victory

CONTAINMENT

When negotiations break down, the prior effort should not be wasted. Both parties have learned more about each other and about areas of mutual interest. Tuckman (1965) describes four stages of human interaction: *forming, storming, norming,* and *performing.* He felt that groups cannot reach the performing stage (i.e., increasing problem-solving ability, exploring new methods to achieve improved outcomes, and inspiring excellence among fellow team members and other teams) without going through the storming stage (i.e., negotiating issues of diversity, control, problem solving, and conflict). It is important to depersonalize potential conflicts by agreeing to talk again in the next weeks or months rather than assigning blame. Discussions may be more favorable after each side learns more about the costs and possible consequences of physician-hospital competition. An orthopedic surgeon described his group's decision to embark on a joint venture with the hospital on an ambulatory surgical center on the hospital campus, writing that the breakthrough came once physicians realized that patients would have been caught in the crossfire between specialists and the hospital (Robinson and Skee 2004). Moreover, referring physicians gain time to make their feelings known to hospital leaders and to physician colleagues considering competitive options. Finally, a time-limited delay may give administrators the chance to prove that they are serious about identifying and removing roadblocks

to effective and efficient processes that waste physicians' time and cost them and the hospital revenue.

Physician conflict-of-interest policies are often a part of these negotiations, but we urge caution in formulating them, as unintended consequences may outweigh their value. Legalistic responses may promote a more adversarial response than necessary; physicians may be considering competitive approaches to reduce inefficiency in the practice environment rather than to harm the hospital. As we will discuss in Chapter 6, hospital executives can lose their jobs when (in the opinion of the board) they lose the confidence of the medical staff. A written pledge from medical executive committee officers and physician board members that they will not use proprietary hospital data to further personal financial interests may be all that is necessary. In the long run, it is less expensive to admit that the hospital will partner in certain circumstances and compete in others than to waste scarce community resources on lawsuits.

The best way for the hospital to be competitive and to retain physician loyalty at the same time is for all of its employees to be focused on delivering outstanding patient care, constantly streamlining policies and processes, decreasing turnaround time, and paring bureaucracy.

Communicating results is another issue that merits attention. Even if some reforms are not possible in the near future, communicating the reasons to physicians may yield valuable information and clarification and help to depersonalize conflict. "Close the loop" should be the mantra of all management meetings; the chief executive officer and chief operating officer can add value by insisting on follow-up to the physicians directly. It is essential for hospital leaders to communicate important information to physicians directly and personally, rather than assuming that physicians will spot the information in a generic form of communication, such as the hospital newsletter.

KEY CONCEPTS

- Complete alignment is a fantasy. Hospital leaders and physicians need effective dialogue to decide where they will partner and where they will compete.
- Being proactive regarding potential collaboration is the best way to keep both parties' expectations realistic.
- When negotiations do not lead to agreement, it is helpful to meet again in future weeks or months to assess progress rather than to blame the other side for failure.
- Streamlined, effective, and efficient processes are the hospital's best opportunity to be competitive and to retain physician loyalty at the same time.
- "Close the loop" should be the communication principle espoused at all management meetings.
- Physicians' entrepreneurial expertise and the hospital's access to capital and technology can open up new markets and enlarge existing markets if both parties remain proactive, pay attention to language and hot-button issues, and act reflectively rather than reflexively.

REFERENCES

Cohn, K. H., S. L. Gill, and R. W. Schwartz. 2005. "Gaining Hospital Administrators' Attention: Ways to Improve Physician-Hospital Management Dialogue—A Case Report." *Surgery* 137 (2), in press.

Gill, S. L. 1987. "Can Doctors and Administrators Work Together?" *Physician Executive* 13 (5): 11–16.

Lussier, R. N. 1995. "Managing Conflict Resolution Models: Five Conflict Management Styles." *Clinical Laboratory Management Review* (January/February): 15–21.

Porter L. 1996. "Conflict." *Seminars in Perioperative Nursing* 5 (3): 119–26.

Robinson, B., and J. Skee. 2004. "Picking Up the Pieces: Physicians Engage Each Other to Optimize Local Care." *Health Care Perspectives* (Summer): 9–10.

Tuckman, B. W. 1965. "Developmental Sequence in Small Groups." *Psychological Bulletin* 63: 384–99.

Umiker, W. 1997. "Collaborative Conflict Resolution." *Health Care Supervisor* 15 (3): 70–75.

Ury, W. L. 1991. *Getting Past No: Negotiating Your Way from Confrontation to Cooperation*. New York: Bantam.

CHAPTER 4

Appreciative
Inquiry

Kenneth H. Cohn, Marianne D. Araujo,

and Sandra L. Gill

A West Coast cardiac surgeon sat down across from me (KC) and crossed his arms over his chest. "As reimbursement drops, the table manners change!" he exclaimed. In a climate of such suspicion, in which he felt his outcomes— over which he had little control except in the operating room—were under increasing scrutiny, how would change be possible? At the time, I mentally dismissed his criticisms as the sin of sophisticated resignation, but months later he and I hit on a more welcoming approach: I asked him if he could remember a time when physicians and hospital leaders had ever worked successfully together. He thought for a moment and mentioned the ongoing collaboration in the cardiac catheterization laboratory. ▶

INTRODUCTION

The purpose of this chapter is to describe the process of appreciative inquiry, which offers an alternative to traditional problem solving and a way to connect with others on the basis of what really matters to them. Although problem solving is an established activity performed at many levels in well-run hospitals throughout the United States, it has side effects and may interfere with change efforts in the following ways (Cooperrider, Whitney, and Stavros 2003):

- Physicians and hospital employees become defensive when hospital leaders view them as problems to be solved.
- Fragmentation and turf battles increase over attribution of blame.
- Negativism and fatigue lead to difficulties with retention and recruitment.
- Response time slows, making it difficult to compete with, for example, ambulatory care centers that offer speed, responsiveness, and care that transcend departmental silos.

AN ALTERNATIVE TO PROBLEM SOLVING

Appreciative inquiry (AI) is a technique that focuses on building on success (Araujo 2003; Ludema et al. 2003). It is based on the premises that people respond favorably to positive reinforcement and that sharing stories of past successes generates more energy and less defensiveness than analyzing problems and attributing blame. The following case study demonstrates the relevance of AI to the hospital setting. (See the appendix at the end of this chapter for a brief guide to the AI process.)

CASE STUDY

At a team-building retreat, a facilitator asked a group of approximately 20 physicians and hospital administrators to remember a time when they overcame differences and worked together. After a brief period of uncomfortable silence, vignettes about the development of the ambulatory surgical center and the recent Joint Commission on Accreditation of

Healthcare Organizations audit surfaced. However, the event that reflected the greatest shared excitement was the response to water contamination while the CEO was out of town. Routine testing showed small quantities of a microorganism, capable of causing systemic illness in immunocompromised patients, arising from an old shower head. Rapid repeat testing confirmed that the results were not caused by any factors introduced in the laboratory and raised the possibility that the hospital water supply might be contaminated. Physicians and management representing infectious diseases; oncology; pediatrics; and the offices of the vice president for medical affairs, patient care services, operations, and public relations cleared their schedules and formed a command post from which they could receive and communicate information rapidly and often. They shut off the existing water supply and made arrangements for an emergency resupply of fresh water from the outside while they researched ways to determine the extent of the contamination, remove the source(s), and purify their water delivery system. They calmly briefed the CEO and board of directors and then employees, the press, and local community agencies to reassure them that they had identified a problem and were in the process of remedying it. In addition, they stepped up the monitoring of susceptible patients. Within three days, they had replaced the old shower heads and purified the water system. No patient morbidity or mortality occurred as a result of the contamination.

Although the departmental culture had created silos that made it difficult to obtain interdepartmental cooperation except in times of crisis, leaving some participants frustrated, all agreed that the shared values, camaraderie, and pride they felt from their rapid and effective handling of a potentially life-threatening contamination episode gave them a sense of accomplishment, on which they could build in the future.

KEY CONCEPTS

- Physicians and senior executives can use appreciative inquiry to overcome defensiveness, turf battles, negativism, and fatigue.
  - Professionals prefer being inspired to being supervised.
  - Usually, it is easier and safer to build on perceived strengths than to tear down perceived weaknesses.
- Storytelling, which is an integral part of appreciative inquiry,
  - decreases the inhibiting effects of hierarchy on an organization,
  - uses metaphors to summarize important points and make them vivid, and
  - provides vignettes that are remembered more readily than facts.

REFERENCES

Araujo, M. D. 2003. "Creating Business Outcomes Through Appreciative Inquiry and the Unconditional Positive Question." Ph.D. diss., Benedictine University, Lisle, IL.

Cooperrider, D. L., D. Whitney, and J. M. Stavros. 2003. *Appreciative Inquiry Handbook*, 272. Bedford Heights, OH: Lakeshore Publishers.

Ludema, J. D., D. Whitney, J. Bernard, and J. Thomas. 2003. *The Appreciative Inquiry Summit: A Practitioner's Guide for Leading Large-Group Change*. San Francisco: Berrett-Koehler.

Appendix:
A Guide to Appreciative Inquiry

INTRODUCTION

- Appreciative inquiry is a technique that focuses on building on past successes rather than on analyzing problems and individual weaknesses.
- It is based on the assumption that people respond to positive approaches.

METHODS

Discovery (Appreciating, Honoring, Valuing)

- Recall a moment when people overcame differences and worked together.
  - What created the positive energy?
  - What did people value about their work, their organization, and themselves?

- How did their level of enthusiasm change?
- How did it feel at that moment to experience what was happening?
- How did the process contribute to the organization's positive core (knowledge, practices, achievements, innovations, values, traditions, assets, capital)?
- Capture the details in a story, written in the first person and told with the breathless, contagious excitement of a child.

Dream (Envisioning)

- What wishes arise from the discovery above?
- If the positive energy were a flame, how would you ignite it?
- How would you keep it burning brightly?
- How would you build on and enhance what happened in the discovery phase?

- Capture the details in bold, positive, uplifting questions that ask, "What are patients (or other stakeholders) asking for? What might they be asking for that we are not anticipating?"
- Questions focus attention, heighten energy, and shift people from acting reflexively to acting reflectively.

Design (Turning the Dream into Reality)

- What are the shared values and principles that the questions build on (design elements)?
- Who are the formal and informal leaders we must reach and involve (key internal and external relationships, dialogue)?
- How do we manage novelty, transition, and continuity (social architecture)?
- How does what we propose fit with our present culture?
- Capture the details in a provocative, affirmative proposition that challenges the status quo, strives for a desirable outcome, and uses widespread participation and external benchmarks.

Destiny (Implementing, Sustaining)

- What will be our future?
- How do we empower, learn, improvise, and adapt?
- How do we build AI learning competency into our culture?
- How do we inspire a movement (vs. making a product)?
- There is no single best way to carry out the destiny phase.

PROCESS

- Continue the ongoing journey through discovery, dream, design, and destiny.
- According to J. Stavros, Ph.D., "Allow yourself to dream, and you will discover that destiny is yours to design" (Cooperrider, Whitney, and Stavros 2003).

Source: Cooperrider, Whitney, and Stavros (2003).

CHAPTER 5

Embracing
Complexity[1]

Kenneth H. Cohn

"There are so many competing interests I don't know how to solve this problem!" exclaimed an emergency department [ED] physician in frustration. "Every time we try to improve patient flow, we run head first into another wall! We expand our ED beds, and then we increase our staff, and then a local hospital closes and we inherit their ED business, and then we run out of capacity on the floors and have to bed patients overnight in the ER..." his voice trailed off. "And we're supposed to be improving our Press-Ganey patient satisfaction scores." He winced. ▶

INTRODUCTION

Understanding principles of complexity science as they apply to healthcare can help hospital leaders relate to physicians and their practice environment. Physicians deal with complexity daily in caring for patients and in working in organizations; yet their training leaves them poorly prepared to deal with processes that they can influence but cannot control (Cohn and Peetz 2003).

The purpose of this chapter is to help administrators and physicians understand principles of complexity science relevant to illness and healthcare organizations. This chapter also clarifies why it is inappropriate to treat healthcare as an assembly line. An assembly line requires predictable, linear, cause-and-effect relationships so that machine operators can limit variation and increase efficiency. Healthcare, on the other hand, is made up of intricate, nonlinear interactions. Knowledge of complexity science can help healthcare professionals understand processes in which many people interact and thus can decrease feelings of helplessness and victimhood.

WHAT IS COMPLEXITY SCIENCE?

Complexity science studies dynamic interactions in living systems and organizations. It is contrasted with linear, mechanical, Newtonian, cause-and-effect systems, which analyze processes by studying their component parts. *Complex adaptive systems* are a collection of component parts or agents, in which individual agents act interdependently so that one agent's response changes the context for all other agents. Real-world examples include the stock market and weather patterns. The only way to know how a complex adaptive system will behave is to observe it. Complex adaptive systems are capable of self-organization in that new structures, patterns, properties, and processes can arise without being externally imposed on the system (Zimmerman, Lindberg, and Plsek 1998). Examples of complex adaptive systems in healthcare include patient flow (discussed below) and human illness. Studying what happens in real-time human interactions can help us make sense of experiences that are neither linear nor predictable and to become more comfortable with processes that we can influence but cannot control.

Glouberman and Zimmerman (2002) define simple, complicated, and complex approaches to demonstrate that interpreting healthcare problems as complex may allow us to have more realistic expectations and more optimism about the current practice environment.

- *Simple problems* are those that we can deal with by following a recipe that promises a similar outcome each time. Simple problems yield a linear, scaleable approach; healthcare scenarios do not fit this category.
- *Complicated problems*, like sending a rocket to the moon, require a high degree of coordination and expertise, respond to learning and knowledge sharing, and offer a high degree of certainty of outcome. A healthcare example might be preparing for a scheduled site visit from a national regulatory body.
- *Complex problems* comprise the majority of current healthcare problems, such as indigent care, risk management, clinical priority setting, and patient flow. Here, formulas have limited applicability and expertise is important, but relationships are key, and doing something once gives no assurance of future success. Dealing with

complex problems requires accepting their uniqueness. An example might be child rearing, where, because of the interplay of genetics and nurturing, raising one child successfully gives no assurance of future success, but people generally remain optimistic.

The advantage of making the distinction among simple, complicated, and complex problems is that issues that seem intractable can be viewed more optimistically and resolved more successfully when examined from a new perspective. Understanding how complexity enters medical practice in patient flow issues and human illness may help physicians and hospital leaders make sense of their experience and work more productively together.

Complex Responsive Processes

Stacey (2003) proposes using the term *complex responsive processes* to describe the way in which communication and power relationships emerge in organizations over time. Stacey writes that organizations are self-organizing patterns of conversation in which human identities emerge. He felt that having formal and informal conversations is an important way that individuals and organizations can deal with complexity. This principle underlies the success of the structured dialogue process described in Chapter 1, where scheduled meetings among physicians and hospital leaders become a forum for formal and informal conversations that can improve communication and hospital processes. Similar principles apply in chapters 7 through 9 of this book, where we discuss engaging physicians in hospital operations, marketing, and identifying early signs of burnout.

Furthermore, Stacey (2003) writes that learning inevitably leads to anxiety because challenges to people's identity are threatening. People cannot know in advance what patterns of identity they are moving into, which may feel like incompetence and failure. In a social order that prizes knowledge and competence and punishes failure, people can feel ashamed about not knowing. Therefore, the challenge facing organizations in times of rapid change is how to create a safe environment for learning (Stacey 1996). For example, a community hospital hosts interdisciplinary conferences called MLEs, or major learning events, because it found that healthcare professionals are more open to discussing improvement opportunities

when they are not giving excuses or trying to cover up mistakes.

PATIENT FLOW

Understanding patient flow requires looking at the entire system rather than the performance of individual units (Brideau 2004). Yet as long as hospital culture remains departmentally focused, interdepartmental cooperation can be more of a nicety than a necessity (Lambert 2004). Quality and safety problems occur in situations in which patient flow is suboptimal, like uncoordinated handoffs in which clinical information is lost; delays occur in instituting life-saving therapy (as when patients are boarded overnight in the emergency department [ED] and do not receive ordered antibiotics in a timely fashion); and patients suffer cardiopulmonary arrest because of missed signs of early deterioration. When caregivers do not trust the system, they hoard supplies and information, making processes even more inefficient. The role of senior leadership is to eliminate roadblocks to and excuses for suboptimal patient flow, giving frontline workers the time, tools, training, permission, and support to create and sustain improvement (Brideau 2004).

Capacity Management

Adding capacity without improving interdepartmental processes has been likened to broadening the wide end of a funnel and expecting flow to improve (Haraden and Resar 2004). At Elmhurst Memorial Healthcare in Elmhurst, Illinois, smoothing the flow of endoscopic elective procedures by capping them at 35 per day and allowing gastroenterologists to see the importance of showing up on time increased productivity to the point that the hospital did not need to build a new endoscopy unit (Lambert 2004).

Coevolution

The complexity science concept of *coevolution* implies that it is impossible to understand systems in isolation (Zimmerman, Lindberg, and Plsek 1998). The following case study is an example of coevolution, in which people and organizations moved forward despite ambiguity, anxiety, and paradox.

CASE STUDY

At Baptist Memorial Hospital in Memphis, Tennessee, a number of rapid-sequence changes were tested in 2002 (Horton 2004). An express admission unit, open 24 hours per day each weekday, resulted in a 50 percent decrease in ED holding hours, as physicians no longer needed to send patients to the ED for workup. Faxing admitted-patient reports from the ED to medical-surgical units decreased time that nurses spent in telephone tag and was a major factor in increasing—from 52 percent to 73 percent—the number of admitted patients who were transferred from the ED to an inpatient bed within one hour of the admission decision. Assigning discharge times for admitted patients prior to their release allowed patients, families, and healthcare workers to work together proactively, helping to decrease length of stay and increase patient and employee satisfaction (Horton 2004).

SURGICAL PREPARATION ISSUES

Pearse et al. (2001) analyzed organizational factors in 159 patients undergoing urgent or emergent surgery in a district general hospital with approximately 180 surgical patients. They found that the preparation of patients for surgery involved more than 20 different staff members. The anesthesiologist recorded the earliest possible time that anesthesia could have commenced and estimated the number of minutes or hours spent correcting organizational problems that were encountered in 54 percent of the patients. Commonly encountered difficulties included the following:

- Laboratory results unavailable (19 percent)
- Surgeon not available because of emergency in another part of hospital (16 percent)
- Patient not adequately prepared on ward (15 percent)
- Transport delay (12 percent)
- Patient eating at time of surgery (9 percent)
- Operating room staff not available (8 percent)

The delays averaged 115 minutes (the range was 5 minutes to 750 minutes). These common organizational difficulties represent latent conditions that may have no adverse consequences but may cause suboptimal outcomes, as when a patient with acute appendicitis was not evaluated by a surgeon for ten hours after arrival in the ED because of a communications mishap. Organizational failures were less common when fewer staff were involved, and patients cared for by a small team during evening, night, and weekend hours had fewer problems than those cared for during regular weekday hours, reflecting better care with fewer interactions.

BUILDING SYSTEMS FROM THE GROUND UP

Edmondson, Bohmer, and Pisano (2001) studied the adoption of minimally invasive cardiac surgical techniques in 660 patients at 16 medical centers to analyze what factors allowed certain teams to learn more quickly than their counterparts at other hospitals, despite completing identical company-sponsored training programs. Success depended on how the teams came together and how they drew on their experiences. Teams that learned new skills rapidly selected individual members based on their ability to work with others, willingness to tolerate ambiguous situations, and confidence in offering suggestions to team members with higher status. High-performing teams emphasized the importance of creating new ways of working together rather than simply acquiring new individual skills. Leaders of successful teams acknowledged the difficulty of the task, emphasized the importance of each team member's contribution, and created an atmosphere of psychological safety so that members felt comfortable making suggestions and trying new processes that might not work. Variations among the teams in educational background and surgical experience, status of the surgeon, support of high-level administrators, and formal debriefing sessions were not significantly associated with shortening the learning curve. This example illustrates the concept of *chunking*, in which team members build systems from the ground up based on the results of past learning and successes (Zimmerman, Lindberg, and Plsek 1998).

CONCLUSION

Collins and Porras (1994) write that visionary enterprises do not simply *balance between* two sets of skills; they *do both* sets of skills. Instead of being oppressed by the "tyranny of the 'or'," these organizations liberate themselves with "the genius of the 'and'." To emphasize their point, Collins and Porras quote F. Scott Fitzgerald: "The test of a first-rate intelligence is the ability to hold two opposed ideas in the mind at the same time and still retain the ability to function." Stacey (2003) defines *paradox* as a state in which diametrically opposing forces or ideas are simultaneously present, neither of which can be resolved or eliminated. It is at the edge of chaos, where both stability and instability are present, that creativity and innovation flourish (Stacey 1996; Zimmerman, Lindberg, and Plsek 1998).

What practical suggestions facilitate success in complex environments? A fundamental principle is that in situations characterized by disagreement and uncertainty, the most important thing that we can do is to learn. Encouraging brainstorming, piloting new ideas, inviting suggestions for improvement, and expecting initial attempts to be a flawed but necessary bridge to future solutions are key to improved outcomes (see sidebar).

Initially, physicians and administrators may be skeptical of complexity science and dismiss it as a fad (Goldberger et al. 2002). The power of complexity science derives from its ability to have us view biological systems and organizations by analyzing their real-time interactions, not just their component parts (Arndt and Bigelow 2000). In

Succeeding in Environments Characterized by High Uncertainty and Disagreement

- Encourage brainstorming and innovative thinking.
- Strive for effectiveness over efficiency.
- Synthesize conflicting ideas with an iterative approach:
  - Act, learn, adapt.
  - "Ready, fire, aim" (i.e., acting without perfect information).
  - Do not expect to get things right initially.
- Reward intuition and muddling through.
- Celebrate learning rather than blaming.
- *Look for improved outcomes rather than ideal solutions.*

times of rapid change, paying attention to human interactions may help physicians and hospital leaders make sense of their experiences and work interdependently in a more productive fashion.

KEY CONCEPTS

- Physicians and hospital administrators deal frequently with complex healthcare problems, such as patient flow, risk management, and clinical priority setting, where relationships are key and doing something once gives no assurance of future success.

- Successful implementation of new clinical programs depends on how well teams work together and on their willingness to tolerate ambiguity and to offer suggestions to team members with higher status.

- Understanding how complexity enters medical practice may help physicians and hospital leaders make sense of their experience and work more productively together.

NOTE

1. Readers interested in learning more about complexity in healthcare may want to visit the Plexus web site at www.plexusinstitute.org.

REFERENCES

Arndt, M., and B. Bigelow. 2000. "Commentary: The Potential of Chaos Theory and Complexity for Health Services Management." *Health Care Management Review* 25 (1): 35–38.

Brideau, L. 2004. "Flow: Why Does It Matter?" *Frontiers of Health Services Management* 20 (4): 47–50.

Cohn, K. H., and M. E. Peetz. 2003. "Surgeon Frustration: Contemporary Problems, Practical Solutions." *Contemporary Surgery* 59 (2): 76–85.

Collins, J. C., and J. L. Porras. 1994. *Built to Last: Successful Habits of Visionary Companies*, 44–45. New York: Harper Business.

Edmondson, A. C., R. Bohmer, and G. P. Pisano. 2001. "Speeding Up Team Learning." *Harvard Business Review* October: 125–32.

Glouberman, S., and B. Zimmerman. 2002. "Complicated and Complex Systems: What Would Successful Reform of Medicare Look Like?" [Online article; retrieved 3/24/04.] www.change-ability.ca.

Goldberger, A. L., L. A. N. Amaral, J. M. Hausdorff, P. C. Ivanov, C. K. Peng, and H. E. Stanley. 2002. "Fractal Dynamics in Physiology: Alterations with Disease and Aging." *Proceedings of the National Academy of Sciences USA* 99 (Suppl. 1): 22466–472.

Haraden, C., and R. Resar. 2004. "Patient Flow in Hospitals: Understanding and Controlling It Better." *Frontiers of Health Services Management* 20 (4): 3–15.

Horton, S. S. 2004. "Increasing Capacity While Improving the Bottom Line." *Frontiers of Health Services Management* 20 (4): 17–23.

Lambert, M. 2004. "Improvement and Innovation in Hospital Operations: A Key to Organizational Health." *Frontiers of Health Services Management* 20 (4): 39–45.

Pearse, R. M., E. C. Dana, C. J. Lanigan, and A. R. Pook. 2001. "Organisational Failures in Urgent and Emergency Surgery: A Potential Peri-operative Risk Factor." *Anesthesia* 56: 684–89.

Stacey, R. D. 2003. *Complexity and Group Processes: A Radically Social Understanding of Individuals*, 297–98. New York: Brunner-Routledge.

———. 1996. "Emerging Strategies for a Chaotic Environment." *Long Range Planning* 29 (2): 182–89.

Zimmerman, B., C. Lindberg, and P. Plsek. 1998. "Edgeware: Insights from Complexity Science for Health Care Leaders." Irving, TX: VHA Inc.

CHAPTER 6

Seven Unhealthy Habits of Hospital Executives

Kenneth H. Cohn and Sydney Finkelstein

"In most doctor–hospital administrator relationships, people talk at each other and not to each other. What each side hears is not what the other side has said at all. They are the definition of a dysfunctional relationship and would benefit from interventional 'marriage counseling'," said a West Coast internist. ▶

INTRODUCTION

The purpose of this chapter is to use a framework (Finkelstein 2003) to focus on ways that physicians and administrators can avoid management failure through efforts with interdependency. Conflict is inevitable in rapidly changing scenarios. Effective recognition and resolution of conflict are key to producing what Hamel (2000) refers to as *creative abrasion*, which leads to innovative solutions, and what Marcus and Dorn (2001) refer to as *metaphorical healing*, which fosters improved relationships.

CASE STUDY

In autumn 2003, the CEO of a 240-bed community hospital lost the confidence of his board and was asked to resign after 25 years at the helm. Although problems had been building for years, conflict between the CEO and the medical staff increased as a result of two events. In March 2002, the CEO replaced the chief of radiology with an outside ultrasonographer to set up a prostate cancer center of excellence, ending a 40-year relationship with the radiologists at the hospital.

Approximately eight months later, the administration refused to recognize the physician-elected chief of staff because of a perceived conflict of interest (the chief of staff had owned a 1.2 percent interest in an outpatient surgery center for the past 12 years) (Rogers 2003). Soon afterward, the board imposed a policy that any physician who has a financial stake in an entity that competes with the hospital cannot hold a medical staff position, be a member of any committee, or vote on any medical staff matter. The hospital adopted a 20-page medical staff code of conduct that gave itself authority to investigate and discipline physicians who did not meet its standards. When the hospital amended medical staff bylaws and took control of the $250,000 medical staff dues fund in spring 2003, the physicians filed suit (Rogers 2003).

"This should be a movie," noted a physician in a battlefield mentality caught up in the distractions of trying to care for patients. A hospital employee characterized the conflict as a "three-dimensional chess game; all of a sudden we were at DEFCON 5 without a clear understanding of how we got there."

The CEO remained defiant. "This is about avaricious, dissident physicians trying to destroy *my hospital*" (italics added), he told a local news reporter (Pezzillo 2003). At a general staff meeting in August 2003, he left the room when he was unable to have the board-appointed chief of staff conduct the meeting rather than the chief of staff elected by the physicians. He was also reported to have tried to unseat elected chairs of several departments and to be associated with administration refusals to make patient charts available for peer review by physicians (Pezzillo 2003).

The elected chief of staff stated, "The code of conduct was put there to get rid of people they didn't want. The conflict of interest [policy] is the same thing. We functioned without those things and we did quite well" (Pezzillo 2003).

The board stepped in at this time and asked for the CEO's resignation. Some participants felt that the board's action was meant to stem the flow of patients to surrounding communities as surgeons moved elective operations to places that they viewed as more welcoming. Yet physicians viewed the CEO's resignation as merely the first step toward healing the strife. "Even if we settled this litigation tomorrow, the hospital will never be the same," noted the elected chief of staff. "Physicians have been vilified,

demeaned, and attacked, and the trust we've had in this institution for so many years has been destroyed. It will take a long time for physicians to feel really secure again and feel like they're here to stay." Another physician concurred, "We know we have a lot of work ahead of us. I'm excited and looking forward to a reversal of these oppressive actions taken by the hospital administration. But we can't afford to become complacent..." (*California Physician* 2003).

Case Analysis

Both administrators and physicians noted that the process went out of control rapidly, a sign that the kindling was very dry and needed just a spark to ignite a conflagration, from which burning embers were evident months after the CEO's firing. Clearly, no administrator seeks to lose support of physicians. Patients generally go to hospitals where their physicians advise them to receive care. It frustrates administrators to be held accountable for the decisions of physicians whom they do not employ regarding revenues, clinical costs, and outcomes. Similarly, it frustrates clinicians who perform procedures to have their incomes held hostage by system glitches and inefficient patient flow, especially when reimbursement does not keep up with rising expenses.

WARNING SIGNS OF CEO LEADERSHIP FAILURE

In *Why Smart Executives Fail*, Professor Sydney Finkelstein (2003) delineates seven patterns that characterize leadership failures at some of the world's largest companies. Analysis of these leadership deficiencies shows that they are not limited to executives of for-profit companies. The personal qualities that make failure possible are often paired with truly admirable qualities, as with the aforementioned hospital CEO who had transformed his organization from a small-town community hospital into a regional center of excellence.

According to Finkelstein, CEOs can exercise great personal magnetism and yet fail—turning modest judgment errors into organizational disasters—because of the following seven habits:

1. *Unsuccessful executives see themselves and their company as dominating their environment.* Such leaders think that they can dictate terms to those around them. They suffer from the illusion of personal preeminence, believing that they are successful because they made it happen. These executives believe that they can create the conditions under which they will operate and can achieve their vision by imposing their will on employees (and physicians whom they do not employ), using intimidation to dominate others. These leaders buy into their image extensively, committing the sin of "sucking their own exhaust," believing that the hype they have generated is true (Finkelstein 2003, 215). People around them fear these leaders' anger to such an extent that they become reluctant to convey any news that might upset their boss, making it difficult for CEOs to learn about issues until they become crises. Such executives may also succumb to the illusion of corporate preeminence: rather than looking to satisfy their customers' needs, they act as though their customers are the lucky ones and their position is invulnerable. The CEO of the community hospital in the case study above lost the confidence of his board when busy clinicians found a nearby hospital that welcomed their patients and their services and, as a result, hospital admissions and revenues dropped.

2. *Unsuccessful CEOs identify so completely with their companies that they lose sight of the boundary between personal and corporate interests*. Chief executive officers are especially prone to overidentify with an organization if they believe that they are personally responsible for its success. They can develop a private-empire mentality, behaving as though they own their institutions and have the right to do anything that they want. They have difficulty acknowledging mistakes because doing so seems like a declaration of personal inadequacy. Such executives may confuse personal adversaries with their institution's adversaries. Just as Stephen Wiggins's hatred of government regulation prevented him from accepting compromises to get on with business at Oxford Health (Finkelstein 2003, 220), so too did the anger of the CEO in the case study make him rail against "avaricious, dissident physicians trying to destroy my hospital" rather than looking to independent physicians for suggestions.

3. *Unsuccessful executives may think that they have all the answers.* Top-notch CEOs dazzle people with their understanding of complex situations and their decisiveness. This talent becomes a weakness, however,

when leaders' need to have the answers prevents them from hearing different points of view and learning new approaches. Such intransigence drives opposing perspectives underground and dampens creativity and innovation. The more such CEOs feel that they can exert power over their institutions, the less they feel that their success rests on circumstances beyond their control. Thus, personal control is both an extension of what they see as their executive role and as protection against their own vulnerabilities. Employees described the CEO in the case study both as a visionary leader and as a micromanager whose desire to control the one group of professionals over whom he had no hiring or firing power led him to impose his own candidates as chief of radiology and chief of staff, starting a battle that cost the CEO his job.

4. *Unsuccessful CEOs ruthlessly eliminate anyone who is not 100 percent behind them.* By defining reformers as negative influences, such CEOs eliminate dissenting viewpoints and cut themselves off from their best chance of correcting problems as they arise. The case study CEO's tenure was marked by a number of job reassignments reputed to have more to do with politics than competence.

5. *Unsuccessful CEOs are consummate company spokespersons, obsessed with company image.* High-profile CEOs who become community leaders may allow media accolades to cloud their judgment and settle for the appearance of accomplishment rather than substantive change. By assiduously cultivating public relations exposure, they raise community expectations beyond what they can meet.

6. *Unsuccessful CEOs underestimate major obstacles, especially if the organization has enjoyed previous successes.* When CEOs become enamored with their vision of what they want to achieve, they may disregard the difficulty of executing their strategy and underestimate the personal and financial costs. When they find that obstacles are more formidable than expected, they tend to escalate their commitment rather than rethink their strategy. Recognizing the point at which escalating commitment is not a viable option may be impossible for the person who made the decision, because pride and self-image are tied up in that decision. Had the case study CEO been able to seek input and accept counsel from a number of independent physicians rather than trying to control them, he might still be working as the hospital's CEO.

7. *Unsuccessful CEOs stubbornly rely on what worked for them in the past.* In a quest for certainty in and control of an unpredictable marketplace, CEOs risk reverting to what has worked for them in the past rather than bringing in new opinions or adopting new scoreboard metrics to assess what is working. Such CEOs fail not because they did not learn but because they learned one lesson all too well. The case study CEO had grown accustomed to achieving his vision by imposing his will on his employees. It may not have seemed like a giant leap to recruit and place physicians according to the same model. After all, he had thrived and won previous battles with other stakeholders.

KEY CONCEPTS

- The seven habits of spectacularly unsuccessful CEOs need to be monitored formally and regularly, especially those of CEOs who think that they know the answers and who underestimate obstacles or rely on past accomplishments.
- Independent, practicing physicians can provide valuable input to the board (e.g., via the medical executive committee)

regarding the seven unhealthy habits because physicians deal directly with patient-care issues daily. Without physician input, the board knows principally only what they receive from monthly management briefings.

- The rationale for physicians and hospital leaders to work interdependently rather than independently is that

- both groups care for the same patients,
- both have complementary insights and valuable experience, and
- the inefficiency of working independently wastes scarce community resources and distracts physicians and hospital leaders from achieving outstanding clinical outcomes together.

REFERENCES

California Physician. 2003. "Ventura Hospital CEO Resigns Post." [Online article; retrieved 2/22/04.] http://www.calphys.org/html/bb401.asp.

Finkelstein, S. 2003. *Why Smart Executives Fail: What You Can Learn from Their Mistakes*, 213–38. New York: Penguin Books.

Hamel, G. 2000. *Leading the Revolution*, 18. Boston: Harvard Business School Press.

Marcus, L. J., and B. C. Dorn. 2001. "Beyond the Malaise of American Medicine." *Journal of Medical Process Management* 16 (5): 227–30.

Pezzillo, B. 2003. "Victory in Ventura." *Southern California Physician* October: 31.

Rogers, C. 2003. "Specialty Hospitals vs. General Hospitals: Healthy Competition or an Uneven Playing Field?" [Online article; retrieved 2/22/04.] *AAOS Bulletin* October: 6–9. http://www.aaos.org/wordhtml/bulletin/oct03/feature1.htm.

CHAPTER 7

Engaging
Physicians in Hospital
Operations

Kenneth H. Cohn and Matthew J. Lambert III

"**W**e're not stupid—we just need to be trained," stated the section chief of general surgery at a community teaching hospital in New England. ▶

INTRODUCTION

The teaching in medical school, residency, and fellowships, which focuses on clinical judgment and outcome skills, minimizes the opportunity for physicians to learn about hospital operations. The rapidly changing healthcare marketplace brings physicians and hospital administrators into close contact. Issues such as patient safety, public reporting, and reimbursement stimulate the need for physician-administration conversation and collaboration. The failure of reimbursement to keep up with rising expenses makes physicians aware of the impact of inefficient processes on their ability to earn income. Clearly, it would be in both parties' best interest to work together more interdependently, but how? The purpose of this chapter is to offer ways to engage physicians in hospital operations, improve patient care, and ensure the viability of hospital and physician practice, as illustrated by the following case study.

CASE STUDY

The medical director of a Northeastern cardiac catheterization laboratory faced a difficult challenge. The proliferation of supplies was creating storage issues as well as limiting the lab's profitability. He knew that closing down a procedure room to add storage space would limit opportunities for future expansion of programs and services. Now that the new information system was coming online, he was being questioned not only about supply costs but also about procedure times and outcomes of his staff of six invasive cardiologists.

Not certain what to do but convinced that ignoring the challenge was not an acceptable solution, the medical director turned to his cardiology colleagues at a staff meeting and asked for their input. He showed simple bar graphs representing average time spent per procedure for each of the cardiologists, who were identified by number rather than name. Only the director knew which name corresponded with each number. The cardiologists agreed that they could see widespread differences. Supply use also was dissimilar among physicians. Data on outcomes like myocardial infarction and death according to American Heart Association category and elective versus emergent status revealed substantial variation. The medical director encouraged the group to share their thoughts in subsequent group meetings on how they might limit variation, improve outcomes, and cut supply costs, telling them that they would reexamine the data in another four months, hoping to see progress. If they could not come to consensus on how to limit variation and improve outcomes and profitability in six months, the director would put names above the individual physicians' numbers and post the data on a bulletin board in the catheterization laboratory in full view of the entire staff.

The medical director's clinical credibility, integrity, and sincerity were unchallengeable. Within four months, procedure times and outcomes for the entire six-person group were within one standard deviation, and the staff had decreased their vendors to two and cut costs substantially, all while improving outcomes. As one of the cardiologists explained, "None of us wanted to be an outlier, except on the positive side."

Case Analysis

Physician leadership can facilitate physician engagement and improvement of clinical outcomes. Nonphysician hospital leaders have a clinical knowledge deficit that they can remedy only by seeking input from physicians and nurses. Institutions

have had success setting capital equipment budgets and allowing a panel of physicians to decide on the relative priorities. It makes sense to involve physician leaders in multispecialty issues such as operating room turnover, on-time starts, and strategies for improving patient flow. As physician leaders increase their understanding of the fragile nature of hospital finances, they can recommend ways to address the high cost of drugs and devices, including speaking to physician colleagues. The following sections offer ideas on how hospital leaders can create an environment and processes that support clinician participation.

FOSTERING TRANSPARENCY

Data Sharing

Most hospitals are not lacking in data. Where they fall short of expectations in practicing physicians' eyes is in the conversion of data to information that can guide practice and improve service and performance.

Therefore, a better place to start than power sharing is data sharing, provided that hospital officials share data in a way that gives physicians a voice. First, hospital leaders need to ask physicians what data they need to care for patients in an optimal fashion. Next, they need to customize the data in a way that makes sense to physicians so that physicians can analyze and assimilate it. Executives should expect initial physician reaction to be critical, especially if the data point to suboptimal outcomes or costs that highlight the role of physicians. The best way to deal with criticism is to invite it with comments such as, "I know that these data are imperfect, and I would appreciate your suggestions on how to improve their accuracy," so that a small group of physicians and hospital leaders can brainstorm together about improvement ideas.

A technique that we have found helpful in engaging physicians in data sharing is to simulate an outcome that exaggerates the presumed inaccuracy, as follows: "So, Doctor, would you say that, because of the way the data are collected, the error rate might be as high as 20 percent (or whatever figure seems appropriate)? Well, even if there were a discrepancy of 50 percent between the actual data and what we collected, the conclusion would still hold. Clearly, we need your help to make the data reporting more accurate. Would you be willing to work with our staff to improve our

data collection processes? In that way, you would have a say in what was collected and how it was reported."

Once a physician is on board, he or she should be the one to present data to fellow physicians, taking advantage of the principle that physicians like to learn from physician colleagues, as long as the presenter has clinical credibility. Therefore, the choice of a physician presenter is significant and should be based on his or her interest and ability and not merely on rank.

If physicians still are unwilling to trust data that hospital officials supply, executives can enlist the assistance of outside agencies to collect, organize, and report hospital data for a relatively modest fee to facilitate conversations on how physicians and hospital leaders can engage in data-driven discussions to improve clinical outcomes.

Respecting Physicians' Time
Healthcare executives can show clinicians that they appreciate their involvement by demonstrating respect for clinicians' time. Even if physicians receive compensation for being a medical director or committee member, the stipend is but a fraction of what a productive clinician can earn by performing patient consultations and procedures. Clinicians' input into

the timing of meetings is necessary, rather than them being told about the timing, even if it means defaulting to a 7:00 a.m. start because later times may conflict with physicians' patient care responsibilities and availability. Meetings should have refreshments, a realistic agenda that outlines what needs to be discussed, and commitment from participants to adhere to the agenda. Each meeting should start and end on time.

Wherever possible, hospital executives should try to remove a task from a busy clinician's plate before asking for assistance with additional tasks. Finally, task force assignments with definite goals and end dates are preferable to committees that take on a life of their own.

Providing Support Services

How support services operate affects physician efficiency and thus is important to clinicians. Physicians need laboratory results in hand when they make morning and evening rounds so that patient care can proceed 7 days per week, 24 hours per day, even if the timing of having access to the results requires adjusting blood-drawing times. The best way to make sure that physicians see new laboratory information is to attach it to the front of the patient's chart, rather

than expecting physicians to look through all of the laboratory values for it. Hospitals with electronic records need to have adequate computer terminals for access and one password for all the different reports, rather than requiring separate sign-in procedures for radiology and clinical chemistry, for example. Allowing remote access from home and office makes it easier for physicians to check in on their patients than calling the floor.

CELEBRATING MILESTONES

It is important to identify interim goals that participants can accomplish readily to obtain quick wins and build on the momentum to tackle more difficult projects. For example, in Chapter 1 we reported that a community teaching hospital successfully implemented improvement efforts, which included decreasing the number of pages physicians received regarding their anticoagulated inpatients (refer to the case study discussion in Chapter 1). Successful joint efforts give participants on both sides a chance to get to know one another as people with families and interests similar to their own and pave the way for future collaboration. Celebrating success at frequent intervals brings participants together and gives them a chance to have informal conversations, which may be key to resolving complexity in the workplace (Stacey 2003).

Paraphrasing the sociologist Emile Durkheim, if people can agree on principles, then all of the laws in the land are unnecessary; if they cannot agree on principles, however, then all the laws in the land are insufficient. At some point after achieving quick wins, it is important for physicians to discuss principles on which they can agree collectively. One of the advantages of a set of written principles is having a document to use in case of infractions and to share during recruitment and orientation, when people tend to be receptive. Knowing that principles will vary in different hospital settings, we offer a few that have resonated at hospitals where we have worked.

- We are committed to delivering outstanding patient care, as measured by acuity-adjusted outcomes and patient and employee satisfaction scores that exceed those of our peer group.
- We are never done; we strive to improve our service to patients on an ongoing basis.
- We treat everyone we encounter with dignity and respect.

KEY CONCEPTS

- Engaging physicians in hospital operations is an important way for physicians and administrators to work together in a more interdependent fashion.
- Possible first steps involve querying physicians on what data they need and then involving physicians in data collection and analysis.
- A few quick wins can help to build momentum and credibility.
- Healthy competition may work with physicians, especially those who do not want to be perceived as negative outliers.

REFERENCE

Stacey, R. D. 2003. *Complexity and Group Processes: A Radically Social Understanding of Individuals*, 297–98. New York: Brunner-Routledge.

CHAPTER 8

What Physicians and Hospital Leaders Can Teach Each Other About Marketing

Kenneth H. Cohn, Audrey S. Wise,
and Dorothy E. Bellhouse

"This hospital does a lousy job of marketing its services," said a disgruntled cardiac surgeon at a large metropolitan center. What frustrated him was that a nearby competing hospital was gaining market share, even though his group had the best outcomes in the state. ▶

INTRODUCTION

Although many physicians may focus narrowly on advertising as marketing or promotion, they also recognize the importance of understanding and meeting or exceeding the needs of patients in their community. Patients often follow physicians' advice regarding where to seek care. The purpose of this chapter is to illustrate, by way of a series of case studies, the importance of ongoing physician-administration and physician-physician communication to identify opportunities for mutual growth and benefit. To promote their services, physicians need to know what services other physicians offer, and hospital leaders can play an important role in facilitating information sharing.

CASE STUDY: "WE HAVE MET THE ENEMY, AND IT IS US"

"How many aortic stent grafts have you implanted fluoroscopically?" barked a usually friendly internist on the medical advisory panel (MAP) of a community teaching hospital as a surgeon finished a presentation on minimally invasive vascular surgery in spring 2000.

"Eleven," replied the surgeon.

"Over how long a time period?" questioned the internist, his voice becoming increasingly tense.

"Four months," replied the surgeon.

"I can't believe it," roared the internist, his fist pounding the table. "I have sent four patients with abdominal aortic aneurysms to an academic medical center in the last two months because I did not even know that we were doing minimally invasive vascular procedures here. We need to do a better job communicating!"

On the strength of the internist's recommendation, physicians now gather quarterly for an evening medical staff meeting; the first order of business is an update on new services. The institution recognized that physician-physician marketing is an important source of hospital referrals, as discussed further in the next case.

CASE STUDY: RESPONDING TO A CHANGED PARADIGM

"It's just not fair," whined a general surgeon during a presentation to the MAP. "We were the first group in the state to perform laparoscopic cholecystectomy, and even though we have all taken advanced laparoscopic courses, we can't get any referrals for the procedures."

A gastroenterologist sitting on the panel responded, "What you don't understand is that times have changed. When you did the first lap choles, there were no fellowship-trained laparoscopic surgeons. Why should we send patients now for laparoscopic procedures to surgeons who have performed them only on pigs, when surgeons finishing laparoscopic fellowships have done more than 100 procedures on human patients? Hire a fellowship-trained laparoscopic surgeon who can train the rest of the general surgeons, and we will be happy to send you patients."

The conversation between the surgeon and gastroenterologist led the hospital to hire a fellowship-trained laparoscopic surgeon on the surgical intensive care unit staff so that private physicians did not feel that the hospital was competing with them. The addition of a fellowship-trained laparoscopic surgeon reversed the flow of referrals back to the general surgeons at the hospital. Discovering and meeting the needs of referring physicians was a win-win situation for the physicians, general surgeons, and hospital. Rapid change is possible when framed in the context of

improving service to patients and physicians, as discussed further in the following case study.

CASE STUDY: INFORMAL SURVEY RESULTS SPUR CHANGE

A survey of primary care practitioners (PCPs) regarding their general surgical needs, conducted in preparation for a presentation to the MAP, revealed a point of dissatisfaction among PCPs who referred patients to surgeons. The patients were returning to their PCP's office for confirmation of the surgeon's recommendations before the PCPs had received letters from the surgeons to whom they had referred their patients. Within 36 hours after the surgeons learned about the PCPs' needs, they began sending faxed recommendations to PCPs the day of consultation, rather than mailing letters to their office.

CONCLUSION

In response to increasing complexity, many physicians have walled themselves off and limited interaction with others to focus on their most pressing tasks. A structured dialogue process gives physicians a forum to reflect on and express their needs. By coming together, they increase their opportunity, through formal and informal conversations, to deal with complexity in a way that improves communication, service, satisfaction, and outcomes in an ongoing fashion.

KEY CONCEPTS

- As with many other personal services, individual patients tend not to think of healthcare until they need it.
  - Physicians and administrators need to keep themselves in the minds of their communities by constantly assessing and responding to the changing needs of potential patients and referring physicians.
  - Only by understanding the needs of their target population can physicians and hospital leaders provide the desired benefits better than their competitors.

- Seeking to establish a branded identity in the current healthcare marketplace is challenging and expensive.
  - Promotion or advertising directed to potential patients should focus on services to which patients can self-refer.
  - For services that require a physician's referral, effective physician-physician communication is essential.

- Language is an important part of the communication process.
  - Words like "patients" and "services" connote long-term relationships to many physicians more than words like "customers" and "products," which have a transactional connotation.
  - Physicians need to feel that they are providing services of value rather than commodities.
  - Physicians, hospital leaders, and patients all benefit when the physicians and leaders treat each other as valued and necessary partners
- Joint presentations by physicians and administrators to interested community organizations build business and promote goodwill and visibility.

CHAPTER 9

Workplace Burnout

Kenneth H. Cohn, D. Bruce Panasuk,
and Jimmie C. Holland

“*I thought that I had my act together until one day I was unable to get out of my car after I parked at the hospital. I sat there for 20 minutes not wanting to go in. Life had gotten out of control,*” *a trauma surgeon confessed at a symposium on surgeon burnout.* ▶

INTRODUCTION

In *Complications: A Surgeon's Notes on an Imperfect Science*, Gawande (2002) writes that even good doctors go bad, and when they do, colleagues tend to be ill-equipped to help. We suspect that burnout involves a continuum of responses ranging from acute exhaustion after being on call during a busy night or weekend to mood swings stemming from the loss of a patient to more chronic symptoms such as impaired performance or suboptimal coping strategies, including disruptive behavior and alcoholism/substance abuse.

Confronting the professional and emotional competence of a physician creates fears that "there but for the grace of God go I"—that we all have dirty laundry that no one wants exposed. The challenge is to identify and intervene in the early stages before patient care suffers. Because burnout has widespread patient safety implications and because it makes so many physicians and hospital leaders uncomfortable, both physicians and executives need to be proactive, timely, and collaborative about identifying and dealing with it. The purpose of this chapter is to describe sources of stress, common symptoms, psychological survival tools, and the need for proactive monitoring of all healthcare professionals, not just physicians.

WHAT IS BURNOUT?

Burnout occurs when work and/or personal demands exceed one's ability to cope; it results in psychological distress, physical symptoms, and/or clinical errors and increased patient morbidity and mortality. The Maslach Burnout Inventory, used to measure burnout, defines it in terms of three components: emotional exhaustion, depersonalization (decreased empathy), and lack of personal accomplishment (Kash et al. 2000).

CASE STUDY

I (DBP) have always looked for the greatest challenge. As a high school and college athlete, I looked forward to competing against the toughest opponents. In medical school, I was attracted to general surgery for the same reasons, drawing inspiration from senior residents and attending surgeons who had the technical ability and the guts—the "clinical courage"—to take on the most complex and demanding cases. I wanted to be that "go to" guy. I pursued a cardiothoracic surgery residency for the obvious reason (obvious to me, anyway): to be with the best of the best, the special forces, of the medical profession. (In fact, during my cardiothoracic surgery residency I was called "Rambo.") If you had told me during residency that in 15 years I would be writing about my own experience with burnout, I would have laughed in your face. Burnout was for the weak.

During the first five to seven years of being in solo practice, I experienced the excitement and novelty of finally being an independent attending surgeon; I was also initially energized by my appointment to associate program director of the general surgery residency. I loved learning, improving my skills, and taking care of patients. I also enjoyed teaching and coaching the residents, being both a role model and life mentor to them. I was good at that. However, almost without my realizing it, the pace of my practice continued to pick up speed. Over the next few years, it became like a runaway train, and being in solo practice made it impossible to control.

Because of the packed schedule together with the constant threat of the pager, everything became a rush. I rushed through rounds, rushed to the office, rushed through office hours, rushed to the operating room, (trying not to rush through OR cases), rushed

home, rushed through meals, rushed through exercise workouts, rushed to get the grass cut, and rushed to spend time with my family because I never knew when the pager would go off. I was on an electronic leash, complete with choke collar. Even when I was watching my children's school activities or athletic competitions, it was hard to be totally engaged because of the burden of the beeper. When the pager went off, I would explode inside, because, once again, someone was taking away my time and pulling me away from my family. To add further to the stress, I was appointed program director of the general surgery residency.

I realized that life had gotten out of control when I helped a resident perform an operation on a patient with esophageal cancer. I remarked that the way he sewed the esophagus and stomach together at the end of the case approached technical perfection and congratulated him on a well-done anastomosis. Two nights later, I was notified that the patient had developed chest pain and died suddenly of a massive heart attack. My immediate thought was, "What a waste of a beautiful anastomosis." The reality of that thought shocked me. Patients and their families did not matter anymore; in fact, they were often obstacles, even enemies. I had to brutally confront the sense of apathy I felt. I wondered, "What have I become?" I had been breaking the speed limit of life, and the law was catching up with me. I had no breathing room, no margin, no reserve. I was physically and emotionally exhausted.

The words of a mentor haunted me: "Beware of what you become while in pursuit of what you want." I had to admit that I had reached a point of burnout. I also recognized that I could not continue the frantic pace of my present practice and simply search for better coping strategies. I had lost my passion and enthusiasm for the practice of surgery, and the erosion was beginning to affect other areas of my life. It was time to wrest control of my life back from the profession of medicine in a radical way. My initial thought was simply to retire from the practice of thoracic surgery. However, my department chair convinced me to take a one- to two-year sabbatical from clinical practice. I could devote my time to the administrative responsibilities of the residency program while regaining control of my life and consider clinical reentry down the road. While I believe he knew that my mind was set about taking a leave of absence from thoracic surgery, he never explored any possible options that might have allowed me to continue clinical activity at a reduced workload. He hired another thoracic surgeon to pick up my clinical activity.

Now, four years later, I am a much happier member of a three-person group of hospital-employed thoracic surgeons, sharing on-call duties, consultations, rounds, and the general office workload. We are able to work this way because we have similar clinical skills, but more importantly, we share similar values of work-life balance and the importance of quality and quantity time with family.

The journey from where I was to where I am now required a huge pushback against a system that rewards producers and turns a blind eye to the consequences until they get out of hand and patients and families suffer. It was like fighting against gravity. I openly discuss Krizek's (2002) article "Surgery…Is It an Impairing Profession?" with residents and anyone else who will listen; I wish that it were required reading for all physicians and administrators. Only rarely do healthcare professionals connect the dots between their personal philosophy and their daily activities. My final take-home message to healthcare executives is, *Do not be content merely to replace physicians. Ask what is going on, and do not just listen to the squeaky wheels.*

SOURCES, SYMPTOMS, AND MANAGEMENT OF STRESSES

Burnout is most often related to a combination of personal and interpersonal stresses, such as perfectionism, long hours, and excessive demands. Common symptoms worth monitoring periodically include a variety of physical and psychological complaints, including sleep and appetite disorders, tension, anger, and inability to experience pleasure from previously enjoyable activities. Measures to deal with workplace stresses proactively include making time to reflect on important issues, participating in educational sessions on campus, and attending meetings outside the medical center with valued colleagues.

THE NEED FOR INSTITUTIONAL MONITORING

It is in the best interests of patients, employees, and healthcare professionals for institutions to take an active role in monitoring and improving the well-being of their workforce. Approaches can be both universal (i.e., applicable to all healthcare professionals) and personal (i.e., customized to each person's needs). The program must be developed with employee input rather than being imposed on them. Handled in a sensitive, confidential, and caring manner, supportive measures can calm anxieties that "big brother is watching" and that monitoring will be used for political purposes. A range of measures can include the following:

- Regularly monitoring team, unit, and individual staff morale via anonymous surveys
- Improving the medical executive committee recredentialing process of physicians to ask physicians how their colleagues and the hospital can help them build and maintain a sustainable practice:
  - Asking physicians to list time spent seeing patients, attending to committee responsibilities, and meeting other administrative and educational demands
  - Letting physicians' colleagues know the recredentialing schedule ahead of time, so that they can provide confidential input
  - Tracking the number of admissions; elective, evening, and weekend operating room

hours; and other case-volume measures

- Providing access to coaching and private counseling, scrupulously maintaining confidentiality
- Ascertaining and remedying the causes of events that result in healthcare professionals losing their temper
- Having a confidential hotline for reporting behavior that has patient-safety or team-safety implications
- Fostering a culture in which healthcare professionals can have lives outside the medical center, celebrating their family and other activities

CONCLUSION

In his address to the graduates of Harvard Medical School, Ned Cassem, M.D., (1979) stated that the best way to survive the demands of residency is to be a "supercoper," advice that is still relevant to healthcare professionals. Because the daily workload involves dealing with unpredictable and often uncontrollable events, he emphasized the importance of peer-group communication and cohesion. In Table 3, we expand on Cassem's ideas to promote well-being in the workplace.

Table 3. Tools to Promote Psychological Well-being in the Workplace

Interpersonal	Intrapersonal
• Watching out for productive, "go to" colleagues, respecting their time off • Sharing feelings with others who have related a stressful event • Showing concern when colleagues exhibit stress symptoms and helping them obtain assistance before patient care suffers	• Sense of perspective and humor (e.g., watching reruns of the television series *M.A.S.H.*) • Vacation • Exercise: aerobic, muscle strengthening, stretching, and deep breathing • Attention to personal hygiene, nutrition, and hydration • Meditation and biofeedback, (bathroom) breaks*, periodic walks • Frequent self-monitoring for symptoms of physical and psychological stress • Seeking counseling when feeling the need to treat symptoms with alcohol or other habit-forming substances • Knowing one's own loss history to understand feelings when a patient who was close to staff dies

* By "bathroom breaks" we mean breaks that do not need to be long but should be frequent; focusing on deep breathing in the privacy of a closed stall helps to relieve chronic stress before it becomes overwhelming.

KEY CONCEPTS

- Burnout involves feelings of emotional exhaustion, depersonalization, and lack of personal accomplishment, most often related to a combination of personal and interpersonal stresses, such as perfectionism, long hours, and excessive demands.

- Physicians and hospital leaders need to be proactive, timely, and collaborative about identifying and dealing with burnout because of quality-of-care and safety implications and because of the importance of rapidly returning healthcare professionals to a state of optimal functioning.

- We all feel uncomfortable probing into areas where we too may harbor dirty laundry. However, if healthcare professionals do not ask proactively about early symptoms of burnout, their reticence may lead to the unnecessary suffering of patients, families, and physicians.

REFERENCES

Cassem, N. 1979. "Internship, Liberty, Death, and Other Choices: How to Survive Life in the Hospital." *Harvard Medical Alumni Bulletin* 53 (6): 46–48.

Gawande, A. 2002. *Complications: A Surgeon's Notes on an Imperfect Science*, 88. New York: Metropolitan Books.

Kash, K. M., J. C. Holland, W. Breitbart, S. Berenson, J. Dougherty, S. Ouellette-Kobasa, and L. Lesko. 2000. "Stress and Burnout in Oncology." *Oncology* 14 (11): 1621–37.

Krizek, T. J. 2002. "Ethics and Philosophy Lecture: Surgery…Is It an Impairing Profession?" *Journal of the American College of Surgeons* 194 (3): 352–66.

CHAPTER 10

What Physicians
and Administrators
Can Learn from
Nurses

Kenneth H. Cohn, Shelley Algeo,
and Katherine Stackpoole

As a 16-year-old, I asked my father, a practicing
neurosurgeon at a community teaching hospital, "Who do
the residents learn from? From you, or from nurses—" He
broke in, "Mainly from me. Only those who are smart
enough learn from the nurses." (KC) ▶

As a nurse, I always said that I would never marry a physician. What I didn't realize, however, was that I would be involved with multiple long-term relationships with physicians (professionally, of course) and that these relationships would require nurturing to succeed. (SA)

INTRODUCTION

All practicing physicians owe a debt to nurses who allow them to be elsewhere, seeing patients, doing procedures, and being with their families while inpatients recover. A California internist remarked, "Nurses are the ones who make you look good." Nurses are the physicians' eyes and ears, providing them with critical patient information. Nurses have stressed the need for more interdependent care for decades. The purpose of this chapter is to incorporate nurses' perspectives into the framework of improving communication and providing more interdependent care.

Interdisciplinary collaboration is key to high-quality outcomes and patient safety (IOM 2004). Therefore, physicians and nurses must manage conflict in a collaborative fashion that strengthens relationships rather than leaving one party feeling intimidated. This chapter is relevant to healthcare executives because they are responsible for and benefit from creating a safe environment for patients and employees.

COLLABORATIVE APPROACHES TO PATIENT CARE

Interdisciplinary Care

In *Keeping Patients Safe*, the Institute of Medicine (2004) reports on two randomized, controlled trials of daily hospital rounds involving all disciplines affecting patient care. The trials, which included more than 1,100 patients, resulted in significant decreases in length of stay, a more favorable perception of teamwork, and a better understanding of the patient care plan. Recommendation 5-6 states that

> Healthcare organizations should take action to support interdisciplinary collaboration by adopting such interdisciplinary practice mechanisms as

interdisciplinary rounds and by providing ongoing formal education and training in interdisciplinary collaboration for all healthcare providers on a regularly scheduled, continuous basis.

We describe an example of such training in the section of this chapter entitled Collaborative Conflict Resolution.

What Hospital Leaders Can Do

Hospital leaders can recognize nurses as the highly trained frontline workers that they are, who deserve to be listened to and accorded respect. Tucker and Edmondson (2003) evaluated nurses at 9 hospitals and observed 166 problems that nurses were required to solve. Of these, 91 percent were classified as system problems because they involved interdepartmental transfers of information or material. These problems caused 8 percent lost time per shift. Although that may seem inconsequential, the dollar cost of 8 percent of a nurse's wages multiplied by the number of shifts and number of floors amounted to more than a quarter-million dollars per 200-bed hospital. The long-term costs of frustration, burnout, and poor retention were significant as well.

Tucker and Edmondson hypothesize that the reason nurses spent 8 percent of their time on problem solving is that 93 percent of that activity was "first-order problem solving," which fixes a problem but does nothing to address the systemic causes. Although nurses feel initial satisfaction from solving problems themselves, chronic first-order problem solving wastes time, prevents leaders from learning promptly about system glitches, and creates problems elsewhere, as, for example, a nurse going to another unit several times for bed linens because her unit ran out.

Administrators, especially unit leaders, who are willing to adopt a different approach, can turn the frustration of system failure into learning and clinical improvement via a three-step process.

1. *Leaders should be available on the floor to field problems*. Nurses were too busy to contact their supervisor for every system glitch, but the unit leaders' availability increased the chances that they learned of the difficulty, investigated the root cause(s), and supported system changes that would decrease the frequency of occurrence. This process represents second-order problem solving.

2. *Leaders should create a safe environment* by inviting floor nurses to express concerns and by admitting their own errors.

3. *Leaders should create and maintain effective processes* by acknowledging frontline nurses' identification of system glitches, following through on their suggestions for improvement, and communicating with people in different departments to implement the suggested changes in real time. We encourage starting with problems that can yield quick wins to build trust and credibility. At establishments like Nordstrom and the Ritz Carlton hotels, which are known for quality service, frontline employees are praised and rewarded for second-order problem solving. Commendation for action sends a message that patient care transcends turf battles.

Hot-button Issues

Both physicians and nurses can benefit from communication techniques that promote trust and feelings of partnership. Nurse educators can be proactive regarding physician-nurse relationships by, for example, instructing all new nurses during orientation on an effective protocol for when to page physicians and what information to have readily available.

Physicians need to demonstrate respect in their exchanges with hospital employees. Having tantrums, throwing instruments, and belittling hospital employees do not promote an environment conducive to safe, effective, and timely patient care. Cordiality and empathy are essential elements of mutually productive dialogue. Nurses do not believe that disruptive physicians are counseled and coached in an effective manner. Formal and informal physician leaders need to take a greater role in addressing the minority who flaunt the rules. Creating a nonhostile work environment transcends bylaws, policies, and procedures and should be the responsibility of all healthcare professionals, not merely those who attend monthly medical executive committee meetings.

COLLABORATIVE CONFLICT RESOLUTION

One of the authors (KS) developed the Taking a Stand program, a comprehensive approach to improving physician-nurse relationships. The process goes beyond code-of-conduct policies and tracking tools to monitor behavior. This program teaches employees (including medical and surgical residents) how to give and receive feedback in conflict situations, which allows them to empathize with others and advocate for their own needs. The four-step model is based on Marshall Rosenberg's (2003) *Nonviolent Communication*.

1. *Observation* (the concrete actions I am observing that are affecting my well-being): "Yesterday, there was a problem with…"
2. *Emotional response* (how I am feeling in relation to what I am observing): "I'm feeling worried and concerned…"
3. *Needs* (my needs, desires, wants; asking for empathy): "Because I need/am depending on…"
4. *Request* (the concrete actions I would like taken in the future; proposing a solution): "In the future, would you be willing to…?"

CASE STUDY

The following scenario highlights the process in which a nurse uses Rosenberg's model to resolve conflict with a cardiac surgeon.

1. *Observation*: "Yesterday, there was a problem with obtaining timely lab results on your patient. I experienced your rage when I reported that the results were not available. I know that you expect your patient's laboratory results to be available by 6 a.m. so that you can form a treatment plan while making rounds and so that I do not interrupt you in the operating room."
2. *Emotional response*: "I feel upset when voices are raised and angry words are used."[1]
3. *Needs*: "Because I need to have a healthy working relationship with you and to solve problems in a collaborative manner."
4. *Request*: "Would you be willing to communicate your needs in a softer tone and join me in meeting with the laboratory supervisor at a mutually convenient time in the future to see how we can resolve this issue?"

Case Analysis
Using the above feedback model changed the situation from one in which a valuable nurse with 15 years' experience considered leaving the profession to one in which the nurse and cardiac surgeon achieved rapport based on mutual respect. Word travels quickly when a nurse is able to address long-standing conflicts head on, which helps other nurses

feel empowered to express their needs in a tactful manner. The end result is an improved patient care environment.

Offensive behavior emerges from the overuse of personality strengths, which go unchallenged by other members of the team (e.g., a surgeon being decisive in the operating room in a situation that does not involve a life-or-death decision may seem oppressive to coworkers). To help both parties depersonalize conflict, the sidebar on page 69 compares generalized outlook and behavior of independent physicians in private practice with nurses who have a more relationship-based outlook, acknowledging exceptions to the general pattern in both groups.

THE NEED FOR TRAINING

Overcoming systemic problems requires a collaborative approach, which often must involve education and retraining. Physicians receive little formal training in process skills (Cohn and Peetz 2003) and thus may resist new approaches. The importance of teaching skills early in residency is clear in the following interchange in which a new intern and an

established nurse collaborated to resuscitate a patient who was acutely short of breath.

I was a new intern rounding on the patients who were signed out to me, and a registered nurse came running out of a patient's room. Waving her arms, she got my attention and directed me toward a room where a patient was having difficulty breathing. The nurse asked very specific and detailed questions of me and carefully followed my orders with respect to procurement of the patient's chart and the patient's old medical history, including medications. This was done while the patient progressed from respiratory difficulty to respiratory distress. The nurse also was clear and successful in transmitting my needs/orders/requests for supplemental assistance, including a respiratory therapist, a code team, and the pharmacy. We were both level headed and clear about our requests of each other. There was no hesitation on either of our parts to address the other's questions or concerns, and we were "in the zone" together.

I feel this interaction was successful because we both trusted each other to focus wholly on patient care. She understood that there was open communication, yet she also did not impede decision making by attempting to take over the management. Her job was as important as mine in that without the link to additional help instantaneously, the patient would have likely stopped breathing. Her care was instrumental to the patient's survival. There were no boundaries of hierarchy, and there was no "fight for control." We both depended on each other to make split-second decisions that were best for the patient, we both trusted the ability of the other without question, and we performed superbly in our defined roles with a successful outcome that would have been impossible without collaboration, communication, trust, and interdependence.

THE ROLE OF HUMOR

Humor, when used tactfully and judiciously, releases tension, provides valuable perspective, and stimulates creativity. In one situation, a nurse walked toward a physician in the hallway and pulled out the laminated feedback card she received during the Taking a Stand program to make sure that she knew the steps required to provide him with feedback. As he saw her approaching, he pulled out his laminated card also. They both began

laughing and were able to discuss their issues in a respectful, noncombative manner.

A Colorado nurse leader coined the term "moan zone" to describe orthopedic surgeons' initial response to any new proposal she put forth. By letting them vent objections and by using humor to empathize with the difficulty of change, she influenced them to accept many changes that they rejected initially, including seeing workers' compensation outpatients within 48 hours of consultation. These changes have improved patient care and hospital compliance with mandatory federal and state regulations.

A director of nursing in Minnesota used humor to diffuse a conflict situation with a spine surgeon, who constantly found fault with the OR staff. The director was asked by the nursing staff to address the surgeon's negative behavior and "get him off our backs." The surgeon, at 6′7″, literally towered over the 5′1″ nursing director. Upon entering the lounge, he began complaining angrily about what was wrong with the OR staff. She interrupted him, saying, "Dr. X, please sit down so we can talk eye-to-eye." (She had to remain standing to make eye-to-eye contact.) He stopped and started to grin, then laughed and sat down. He became affable, and they discussed what he needed, how the OR staff could help, and what he might do differently when dissatisfied. From that day on, he remained gracious and friendly, and the staff stopped complaining about his behavior.

KEY CONCEPTS

- System glitches aggravate everyone, not just physicians.
- Reframing healthcare workers' perceptions of system failures from sources of frustration to sources of learning allows hospital leaders to engage employees in system improvement efforts that would not occur otherwise.
- Allowing nurses to see their feedback result in changed processes affirms their worth as valuable frontline employees who spend more face time with inpatients than do physicians and administrators and thus have important insights to offer.

NOTE

1. We include a statement about the importance of sending "I feel" messages rather than "you make me feel" messages and of using "and" or "at the same time" rather than "but." "You" messages and "but" tend to encourage defensive reactions and resistance rather than collaboration (Cohn and Peetz 2003).

REFERENCES

Cohn, K. H., and M. E. Peetz. 2003. "Surgeon Frustration: Contemporary Problems, Practical Solutions." *Contemporary Surgery* 59 (2): 76–85.

Institute of Medicine (IOM). 2004. *Keeping Patients Safe: Transforming the Work Environment of Nurses*, 361–63. Washington, DC: National Academies Press.

Rosenberg, M. B. 2003. *Nonviolent Communication: A Language of Compassion*, 2nd ed. Encinitas, CA: Puddle Dancer Press.

Tucker, A. L., and A. C. Edmondson. 2003. "Why Hospitals Don't Learn from Failures: Organizational and Psychological Dynamics that Inhibit System Change." *California Management Review* 45: 55–72.

CHAPTER 11

Orientation:

Another Opportunity to
Engage Physicians

Kenneth H. Cohn

"**W**hy aren't we doing a better job orienting our new docs?" asked the CEO of a tertiary care hospital in Colorado. "It seems like the perfect opportunity to communicate expectations and to socialize new recruits." ▶

INTRODUCTION

After hearing the CEO's query (see beginning quote), I volunteered to learn more and report back to him. I met with approximately 30 administrators who worked daily with physicians and asked them for their impressions of orientation. Most of their impressions were negative as well. I asked them to write the most important parts of orientation on Post-It-type notes, which we spread out over a blank wall. We reflected on what we had contributed and rearranged some notes, which I summarized on a one-page diagram.

When I showed the diagram to the CEO, he was stunned to see that orientation was so multifaceted that nobody could monitor, control, or own the entire process. His chief nursing officer pointed out, however, that individual employees could own certain steps and that by assigning roles or by asking for volunteers and mentors, it might be possible to improve the process to everyone's benefit. For example, the CEO could share stories about the hospital's mission, vision, and culture (see Figure 3). Members of the department or section could provide job-specific information. A mentor could answer basic questions and participate in

reverse mentoring; that is, new recruits could describe and teach approaches used at their previous institutions. During this process, we realized that although orientation was multifaceted, it embodied a series of processes that could be studied and improved. We learned that orientation needed to begin during recruitment rather than when a new recruit was expected to begin seeing patients.

Recruitment is an elaborate courting ritual in which both physicians and hospital leaders are eager to make a positive impression. It also represents an ideal time to begin the orientation process. The purpose of this chapter is to describe how tasks are accomplished in the hospital system, job-specific roles, and personalized aspects of orientation.

HOW TASKS ARE DONE

As illustrated in Figure 3, a systemic approach to orientation represents an opportunity for leaders to use anecdotes to explain to new recruits the organization's mission, vision, values, and culture—the elements of the past that shape the organization's approach to present and future issues. Because most physicians lack knowledge about hospital finance, the

Figure 3. A Systemic, Proactive Approach to Physician Orientation

Orientation
Making people feel that they made the right choice

System — How we do things	Personal — Creating a great first impression	Job-specific — Helping new hires to feel productive and happy

Mission
Vision
Values
Culture
Expectations
• employee
• management
Finances
• operating budget
• capital budget
Quality/safety
• improvement
• credentialing
• accreditation
• continuing medical education
• recertification
 	
General processes
• orders
  –medications
Information services
• training
• customization
	Human relations
	• parking
	• benefits
	• photo ID
	• notify other workers
	Spouse orientation
	• MD spouses
	• community volunteers
	• meet employees (e.g., CEO)
	Mentoring
	• partners
	• medical director
	• unit director
	  –tasks/ telephone numbers
	• emotional intelligence/
	
	leadership training
	• ongoing communication
	• mentee becomes mentor
	Proactivity
	• preventing crises
	• identifying goals
	• aligning with vision
	• helping new hire succeed
	• becoming employer of choice
	• decreasing voluntary turnover
		Specific processes
		• orders/ medications
		• documentation
		• dictation
		• task forces
		• process-skill training
		  –communication
		  –team building
		  –negotiation
		  –conflict resolution
		• peer review
		• chart review
		• outcomes
		• quality improvement
		• service excellence
		Service line
		• scope
		
		• scale
		• goals, roles, expectations
		• trends
		• forecasts
		• marketing
		• performance monitoring
		Meeting other stakeholders
		• patients and family
		• community organizations
		• suppliers
		• physicians
		  –referring
		  –consulting
		Meeting employees
		• formal leaders
		• informal leaders

Building an environment that facilitates two-way communication
Developing transparency, trust, and credibility

Analyzing strengths, weaknesses, opportunities, threats   Setting strategy
Building on strengths   Implementing strategy
Determining priorities   Obtaining results

recruitment stage is an ideal time for giving physicians basic information about sources of revenue, expenses, and the capital budgeting process, which can lay the groundwork for realistic expectations and help prevent feelings of mistrust later.

Administrators can also impart information about quality and safety issues; recredentialing; federal, state, and local regulations; and expectations regarding collaboration and the avoidance of hostile work environment complaints.

JOB-SPECIFIC ROLES AND RESPONSIBILITIES

Another important aspect of orientation centers on how the new recruit will interact with others in the department or section. Here is a chance for physicians to meet members of their team and come to consensus regarding goals, roles, and expectations. It also is a good time for physicians to begin learning about the needs of others, including patients, families, nurses, consulting and referring physicians, and vendors. Finally, orientation is an opportune time to discuss and rehearse specific processes, such as new surgical procedures, and to gain an understanding of relevant quality and safety issues (and the roles of people and committees whose action affects new physicians) before physicians begin seeing patients.

PERSONALIZED ASPECTS OF ORIENTATION

The previous two sections of this chapter involve information transfer mainly from hospital executives and team members to new physicians. In the context of personalized aspects of orientation, the process should be reversed as people in the hospital welcome new recruits and their family to the community; identify potential process improvements and roadblocks; and determine and provide the key factors necessary for success, including contacts, mentors, and supplies. When hospital employees provide a nurturing environment, they not only create a positive first impression but they also help new physicians feel that they have made the correct decision to work at their new hospital.

KEY CONCEPTS

- Adopting a systemic, proactive approach to physician orientation may improve recruitment and retention.
- Placing all relevant orientation processes on a one-page diagram helps hospital employees understand and take ownership of individual steps of a process that is too large for anyone to own in its entirety.
- A visual diagram also helps process owners to see how their roles fit into a larger perspective and to track overall progress.

Afterword

The three principal concepts in this book are that

1. promoting effective communication is in both physicians' and hospital leaders' self-interest;
2. obtaining quick wins in streamlining processes and improving operations is crucial to building momentum and credibility; and
3. responding to nonurgent questions with, "I'm not sure; what do you think?" is an underused way to bring in fresh approaches and energy.

Promoting effective communication. The phasing out of cost-based reimbursement has made it impossible for physicians and administrators to pass on costs independently of one another. Regulatory scrutiny and the wave of consumerism also have increased interactions between physicians and healthcare leaders and have fostered a need for working more interdependently. Yet the financial and time pressures of the current healthcare marketplace make it difficult for physicians and administrators to reflect and have meaningful conversations with one other. The structured dialogue process, in which a panel of respected clinicians recommends clinical priorities for the next three years, creates an ongoing forum for open and effective dialogue between physicians and hospital leaders. Financial collaboration based on effective dialogue also can increase physicians' sense of ownership and create an enterprise of value that benefits patients, physicians, and the hospital.

Appreciative inquiry builds on past successes, avoiding the defensiveness and resistance to change of more traditional problem-solving approaches. The storytelling approach, a component of appreciative inquiry, provides vignettes that are more memorable than facts or sermons. Complexity science studies interactions in living systems and thus offers a scientific approach to analyzing interdependence in the human body and in healthcare organizations.

Obtaining quick wins. A few quick wins can prove to skeptics that hospital leaders are eager to share data, streamline processes, and improve patient care. Operations and marketing represent opportunities for collaboration based on shared self-interest. Similarly, knowledge gained from closer attention to the early stages of burnout may help staff share concerns and mitigate patient safety issues.

Seeking others' opinions. Physician-nurse collaboration is key to obtaining high-quality clinical outcomes and to maintaining patient safety. Allowing nurses to see their feedback result in changed processes affirms their worth and improves patient care. Similarly, adopting a systemic, proactive approach toward physician orientation can facilitate recruitment and retention.

CONCLUSION

Promoting effective communication, obtaining quick wins, and seeking others' opinions are merely the beginning of a lifetime journey. In writing this brief book, I hope to stimulate discussion and to make healthcare professionals excited to be integral parts of our dynamic, challenging healthcare enterprise.

Suggested Reading List

Brideau, L. 2004. "Flow: Why Does It Matter?" *Frontiers of Health Services Management* 20 (4): 47–50.

Cooperrider, D. L., D. Whitney, and J. M. Stavros. 2003. *Appreciative Inquiry Handbook*. Bedford Heights, OH: Lakeshore Publishers.

Finkelstein, S. 2003. *Why Smart Executives Fail: What You Can Learn from Their Mistakes*. New York: Penguin Books.

Gill, S. L. 1987. "Can Doctors and Administrators Work Together?" *Physician Executive* 13 (5): 11–16.

Krizek, T. J. 2002. "Ethics and Philosophy Lecture: Surgery...Is It an Impairing Profession?" *Journal of the American College of Surgeons* 194 (3): 352–66.

Larson, L. 2002. "Balance of Power: Encouraging Physicians to Help Set the Strategic Plan." *Trustee* September: 13–17.

Marcus, L. J., and B. C. Dorn. 2001. "Beyond the Malaise of American Medicine." *Journal of Medical Process Management* 16 (5): 227–30.

Rosenberg, M. B. 2003. *Nonviolent Communication: A Language of Compassion*, 2nd ed. Encinitas, CA: Puddle Dancer Press.

Tucker, A. L., and A. C. Edmondson. 2003. "Why Hospitals Don't Learn from Failures: Organizational and Psychological Dynamics that Inhibit System Change." *California Management Review* 45: 55–72.

Ury, W. L. 1991. *Getting Past No: Negotiating Your Way from Confrontation to Cooperation*. New York: Bantam.

Zimmerman, B., C. Lindberg, and P. Plsek. 1998. "Edgeware: Insights from Complexity Science for Health Care Leaders." Irving, TX: VHA Inc.

Acknowledgments

Although this book is my first, I cannot imagine writing any book alone. I owe my coauthors a tremendous debt for their insight and willingness to share their experience. I accept responsibility for any errors or misstatements, but they deserve the credit for giving each chapter its ability to stand alone and for making this book far better than anything that I could have written on my own. I thank Tom Allyn, Glenn Cordner, Jim Dorsey, and David Sundahl for "volunteering" to read the book in its entirety and for providing me with feedback on a tight deadline. I thank Jim Taylor for help with the complexity chapter; John Miller and Liz Lewis for their ideas on hospital operations; Linda Rusch and Marney Halligan for their input on the nursing chapter; and my partners at Cambridge Management Group—Bob Harrington, Jim Dorsey, Steve Mirin, and Andy Nighswander—for their help and encouragement, especially with the chapter on structured dialogue. Sharon Hogan provided invaluable assistance in crafting the book proposal. My editors, Audrey Kaufman and Joyce Sherman, gave me the ideal blend of distance and support that allowed the manuscript to progress from fantasy to reality.

While writing this book, I neglected all of my family responsibilities; my family richly deserves this book's dedication.

About the Author

Kenneth H. Cohn, M.D., FACS, is a board-certified general surgeon, currently splitting his time between providing *locum tenens* surgical coverage in New Hampshire and Vermont and working as a consultant at Cambridge Management Group, which specializes in physician-physician and physician-administration communication issues. Before obtaining his MBA from the Tuck School of Business at Dartmouth College in 1998, Dr. Cohn was associate professor of surgery at Dartmouth-Hitchcock Medical Center and chief of surgical oncology at the White River Junction VA Medical Center. Dr. Cohn received his medical degree from Columbia Medical School in New York.

Dr. Cohn's father was a neurosurgeon, and his mother taught art and is still active in philanthropy. From their example, he learned the values of service, integrity, passion, and humor.